ARE YOU REALLY OK?

ARE YOU REALLY OK?

ROMAN KEMP

With Susanna Galton

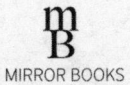

MIRROR BOOKS

To Joe, of course.
And to my mum, who saved me.

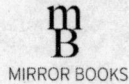

MIRROR BOOKS

Copyright © Roman Kemp 2023

The right of Roman Kemp to be identified as the owner of this work has been asserted in accordance with the Copyright, Designs and Patents Act, 1988.

All Rights Reserved. No part of this publication may be reproduced, stored in a retrieval system, or transmitted in any form, or by any means, electronic, mechanical, photocopying, recording or otherwise without the prior permission in writing of the copyright holders, nor be otherwise circulated in any form of binding or cover other than in which it is published and without a similar condition being imposed on the subsequent publisher.

1

First published in hardback in Great Britain and Ireland in 2022 by Mirror Books, a Reach PLC business.

www.mirrorbooks.co.uk
@TheMirrorBooks

ISBN: 9781915306531
Hardback ISBN: 9781914197512
eBook ISBN: 9781914197529

Written with Susanna Galton.

Photographic acknowledgements:
Roman Kemp, Global Media & Entertainment Ltd, Reach Plc.

Every effort has been made to trace copyright, any oversight will be rectified in future editions.

Design and production by Mirror Books.
Editing and production: Paul Dove, Harri Aston, Adam Oldfield.

Printed and bound by CPI Group (UK) Ltd,
Croydon, CR0 4YY.

CONTENTS

Part 1

Joe, Me and You:
Sharing Saves Lives 1

Part 2

It's All In Your Head:
The Big List Of My Life 18

#1 Babydom 20
#2 School Days 24
#3 Teenage Kicks 30
#4 Dad 39
#5 Mum 46
#6 Girls And Love 51
#7 Family Matters 64
#8 Work 75
#9 Music 98
#10 Exercise 105
#11 Food 108
#12 Sleep 114
#13 Mates 117
#14 Money 121

CONTENTS

#15 Tattoos 127

#16 Drink And Drugs 130

#17 My Phone 138

#18 Dogs 144

#19 Laughter 147

#20 Religion 151

#21 Football 154

#22 The Royal Family 167

#23 Telly 173

#24 Holidays 183

#25 Cars And Travel 189

#26 Home 194

#27 Fame 198

#28 My Godfather 204

#29 Lockdown 213

#30 Radio & Back To Joe 216

Part 3

My Darkest Hour
And Brighter Days To Come 232

The End Of The Book:
Stuff That's Good To Know 256

Thanks

I've been told that you should include an acknowledgements section in books. A bit like the credits at the end of a Netflix drama that you never really read.

Well, I'll keep it short and sweet. Thanks to everyone who has helped me. You know who you are and you know how grateful I am for what you do.

Now let's get on with the book. I hope you get something from it.

Roman

JOE, ME AND YOU

PART 1.

Sharing Saves Lives

I never intended to write a book. I'm a 29-year-old guy and I always thought writing a book was something older people did at the end of their careers. What have I got to say for myself?

In fact, I'd put money on my old teachers saying I would be the last person at school to ever sit down and write a book. I wasn't exactly academic growing up. I was always the class clown, constantly showing off (if I wasn't busy playing with my hair and my trusty GHD straighteners) and entertaining my mates, normally with impressions of all the teachers.

My dad, Martin Kemp – the former Spandau Ballet bassist and EastEnders actor (you may know him) – wrote an autobiography which I did read. But the one he and my mum, Shirlie – who was a singer with Wham! and Pepsi & Shirlie in the 1980s – wrote about their love story… well, being totally honest, I've never actually read it.

But while I'm not much of a reader, when it comes to talking, that's something I can do. Which is fortunate, because as a radio DJ for Capital FM that's exactly what I spend my time doing, it's how I earn my living and I've always been very comfortable doing that, as well as being in front of the camera.

I've never wanted to coast along in life just because my parents are famous, that whole idea just makes me cringe. I've grafted to be where I am, and quite right too, so I should have. Life is tough, and no one deserves an easier ride or special treatment because of who their parents are.

But then, in the pandemic, something terrible happened. And it turned my whole world upside down. My best mate – and the producer who was constantly by my side, who taught me everything about my radio career from the very start – took his own life.

Joe was just 31, a good-looking boy, hugely talented, and

one of the funniest people on Earth. He had his whole life ahead of him – and big dreams with what he wanted to do with it.

His sudden and completely shocking death was far, far worse for his loving, devoted family than it was for me of course. Their deep loss isn't mine to 'steal'.

Yet, my God, was I left reeling from it. Shocked. Confused. Fucking furious at him. I felt utterly horrified and sick to the stomach that I'd had no idea he was so unhappy. I spent all my working hours with him, sitting two feet apart. I hung out with him most nights and weekends too. How could I not know how bad he felt? How could I have let him down? I just wanted my mate back.

Joe's death changed everything.

I became obsessed with suicide, something I'd never have predicted. Because, until Joe, I was lucky enough not to have been directly touched by it, and not to have wholly grasped the complete destruction it leaves in that person's wake.

Losing Joe made me start researching how many young men take their own lives every year. And the answers shocked me.

Suicide is the single biggest killer of men under the age of 40 in this country.

Why? Why is this the case? And why, therefore, is there still so much shame surrounding human beings choosing to take their own lives?

Often, people don't even like to say the 'suicide' word out loud, they might whisper it, or perhaps mouth it instead. Like it's dirty. It's a bit like how the characters in the Harry Potter books can't bring themselves to say the name 'Voldemort' because even the word scares them shitless.

The truth is, we are all terrified and deeply ashamed of talking about our mental health. The dark place our own minds can take us to is scary. We are all guilty of seeing it as a weakness to not be 'fine', to feel it's somehow unmanly to not feel 'OK'. Even though, truthfully, how many of us don't suffer from feeling crap sometimes? How many of us feel like we're not actually coping? How many times a day do each of us shrug off that simple question 'how are you?' with a nonsensical, automatic reply, 'Yeah, I'm fine mate, you?'

When I started looking into it closely, I learned that more than three-quarters of men feel they can't confide in those closest to them about their problems.

But until we confront this big problem, of driving our real feelings underground until we are truly honest and own those feelings, we cannot get rid of that stigma. And even more young lives will continue to be lost. Senselessly lost.

We have to change that as a society.

So I decided I would write a book after all. And I'd put my name and my face out there in the open.

I know that through my radio show, and from being on TV, and yes, OK, because of who my family are, I know I have a platform. And it matters that I put that platform I am fortunate enough to have to good use.

If me opening up saves just one guy – or girl – from taking their own life, it's worth it.

So I'm sharing my story, warts and all. I'm unpacking here for you all the random stuff that goes round in my head, because it's all these bits and pieces – some significant and some seemingly silly – that make me who I am.

With any luck there'll be a few moments that will make you laugh along the way. I promise it's not all heavy going or doom and gloom…!

But I hope that by talking honestly and openly about my life, other young guys like me, guys like the ones you might know, and live with and love, might feel like it's OK to speak out about how they really feel too.

Even if it's not good. Especially if it's not good.

I want to get people talking. I don't want kids to grow up feeling ashamed if they're having a bad time. I don't want young men to feel their only way out, their only way to find calm and peace, is to end their own lives. I want us all to check in on each other. Like, *really* check in.

Asking not once, but twice… "Are you *really* OK?"

Let's get rid of this secrecy about mental health once and for all.

It breaks me that I wasn't there for Joe. I want people to be the hero to their friend that I wasn't to mine.

Tuesday, August 4, 2020:
A waking nightmare

About once a week I give talks about Joe, and about his death, to all sorts of organisations and businesses, and all the funds go to Joe's Buddy's Line – a charity set up by Joe's family to provide mental health workshops in schools, and for the provision of a range of other, crucial mental health initiatives.

And I feel it's my duty to share with you here what I have learned about suicide – in case it can help someone you love, too.

Because this mission I'm on all started with Joe's death, I should first fill you in on how it unfolded.

It is August 2020. The pandemic has been raging for several months, and the day starts just like any other during that weird first summer, when the world is adjusting to the new normal.

Waking up at the crack of dawn, blackness still outside. I go through my automatic morning routine – shower, pulling on clothes, eating porridge, taking my sertraline.

I head to the radio station – I'd started cycling there in the pandemic – and it looks like London is in the middle of a zombie apocalypse. The roads are so beautifully empty. The journey takes about 10 minutes.

When I get into the building, the first thing I notice is Joe isn't there. Normally it's me who is the last one there. I'm always late. The rest of the team, eight or nine of us, are all there, busy prepping for the breakfast show.

We're a tight bunch. Talking to each other non-stop. We've all seen each other angry, sad, happy, sharing those big life moments you do as colleagues. When you work closely like we do, and on a live show, you become a little family. You see each other more than your own family, in fact.

And at the heart of that family there was always me and Joe. We were the duo that it all grew from.

We go on air at 6am, so at five minutes past, I text him. 'Let me know you're OK mate.'

He's obviously overslept.

I'd seen Joe at work the day before and he was fine. And just that weekend we'd hung out and watched football together, and had dinner with my parents at a local restaurant. Typical stuff.

Mum remembers watching us both walk away after that meal to go out in Soho, feeling so pleased I was with Joe. As a parent, she says, you worry who your kids are hanging out with, who they're drinking with, whether they'll get home safely. But she never had concerns with Joe. She felt safe when I was with him because he was just that kind of lovely, sorted human being.

It wasn't unusual for someone on the team to be late

– someone's fallen asleep, or is hungover. We're a young team. That's not unheard of. For a 30-year-old guy not to be somewhere at 5am isn't exactly abnormal, is it? So we all kind of laugh, speculating about where Joe is.

Joe was dating a lot, he was always full of funny stories. I think – he's gone out, gotten drunk, ended up at the girl's house, and he hasn't charged his phone. Classic scenario.

I imagine him waking up with no battery, and doing what we call 'the panic dance'. You know that thing when you wake up late and you're not coming or going or achieving anything? You're dancing around in all directions, like a crab, not sure what you should do first.

He'll be here in an hour, I tell myself. Then I can really rinse him.

Someone tries to call him but it goes straight to voicemail.

I think, 'he's going to be so angry when he wakes up and realises his phone is completely dead'.

That day I start the show, feeling a bit weird not having him next to me, where he has been for every show for the past five years. But I merrily chat away on air, playing Ed Sheeran, Justin Bieber, Harry Styles. Standard Capital fare.

I'm joking and laughing but a little niggle is setting in. I love that boy, and I know he'll be massively stressed about being late. He's a professional.

We decide someone should go and wake him up. Joe doesn't live far away, he shares a flat with his sister Lou in Camberwell. It can be cycled in minutes.

We contact his sister, but she says she hasn't been at home that night and wasn't in the flat herself.

It's the gap between 7am and 7.30am when the mood changes from being jokey to feeling worried.

'Have you heard from Joe?' I text Matt and Charlie. My two best mates from school have become Joe's great mates over the years too. They haven't either.

I can't go to his flat myself, I'm on air. So our executive producer sends another producer, she's also a great pal of Joe's, to go and knock for him.

Where I sit at work, there is a glass panel to my left. And I can see straight down the corridor to our table where my team sits, so from 7.30am to 8am I'm constantly glancing over to see what's going on.

Three of us, me and my co-hosts Sonny Jay and Sian Welby, are all doing the same thing. We can see there's activity going on. We're exchanging looks but we're chatting away, filling the space between songs.

Joe was always a bit careless about leaving his front door unlocked. So despite no one answering the knocks, our producer is able to get in the house.

And from my seat I can see how the vibe in the office has changed.

There seems to be a state of panic, everyone is on the phone to someone else. Something is kicking off.

Something serious has happened.

I stick a song on and march over to the executive producer outside the studio.

'What's going on?' I demand, there's a feeling in my stomach like a knotty kind of dread and fear. 'What's happening?'

The second I saw her face, I knew.

She's in a state of shock. Pure shock. Her eyes are wide, her whole body is visibly shaking… she doesn't need to say anything.

'He's gone, hasn't he?' I say, feeling complete disbelief that those words are coming out of my lips.

She just nods. 'Yeah.'

What comes next is a sort of blur, people burst into tears, there's some screaming I think. Sonny is crying. I stare at him, abstractly thinking, 'I've never seen you cry before.'

I don't cry. Not yet.

I go into a real protection mode over the team. There is still an hour and a half to go of the show. Just music is played, and someone else is drafted in to take over at 9am.

The listeners are confused, people are speculating on Twitter – what has happened on Capital?

We all stay in the office, not knowing what to do with ourselves.

No part of me imagines at this stage that Joe has taken his own life. Your brain goes into overdrive coming up with the most plausible imaginary scenarios.

I genuinely think he's choked on one of his beloved fried chicken wings he's always eating. Or I wonder if he's banged his head in the shower hungover. It's all been a terrible accident.

Poor, poor Joe. I hated the thought of him being alone and frightened and choking.

I ring Mum and Dad, my first port of call in any crisis. They are just waking up.

'Joe's died,' I blurt out to my mum. It's the first time I say it aloud. It doesn't feel real.

I hear her scream and then my dad in the background. 'What's happened?'

'I think he choked on something,' I say.

Dad is crying too, and just saying how cruel it is, how he doesn't deserve this.

Despite my shock, I go into some weird autopilot work mode, trying to make sure the others are OK. I feel responsible for them, like I need to take charge. But the office has become stifling. We go up on the building roof for some air.

'We'll get through this,' I tell them, having no real idea how. 'We'll figure out what happened.'

When we do find out what happened, of course, we are left reeling even more.

The producer who had gone to find Joe had seen he wasn't in bed and the bathroom door was shut. There was something behind the door, and she couldn't open it.

She'd rung the police and the ambulance. She'd eventually forced her way inside the bathroom. And she'd sat with Joe there, holding his hand for the 20 minutes until the emergency services arrived. I'll always love her for doing that. She'd just lost one of her best mates, but she didn't want him to be alone.

When it finally became apparent that Joe's death has been from suicide… well, God. I don't even have the words to describe how I feel.

The all-consuming shock was still there. Yet I went from feeling so, so sad that something had happened to him, an accident, and that he'd been frightened and alone… to being so, so angry.

How could he?

I felt lied to. How could I not have known he was in this much pain?

He lived minutes away from me, I could have cycled there, been there. Stopped it from happening.

Over the next hour or so, everyone numbly congregates back at my flat. We don't know what to do. We don't know where to go. We don't know what to say. But our instinct is that we need to be together. I just want to gather everyone up and close to me.

SHARING SAVES LIVES

All the team from work, Mum and Dad, my sister Harley, my oldest mates Charlie and Matt, they all come to my flat in various states of a daze. Mum makes herself busy pouring mugs of tea for people.

We sit in silence, mainly. On my sofa, forming a sort of circle. Trying – and failing – to make any sense of what has happened. Outside there is beautiful sunshine, which just feels so wrong. So surreal.

When we are all together, I can finally let go of all the emotion and confusion of the past few hours.

I hold Charlie and just cry and cry into his shoulder.

There are journalists trying to find out what has happened, but because the police are involved, there has to be an investigation. We aren't allowed to talk about what's happened to anyone outside.

I think of Joe's family, having to be told by the police that their bright, brilliant – beloved – son has passed away. It's too much to bear, imagining his mum.

I go into my bedroom and sit down on my bed, knowing I have to go through the phonebook, telling all the people we know the awful, awful news that our friend has gone. 'Joe's dead.'

Hearing everyone's shocked reaction, again and again, was heartbreak after heartbreak.

I don't sleep that night. People offer to stay with me, but I need to be alone. When everyone leaves, I just want to speak to Joe.

I feel he might come to me in a dream, or a vision, that's what I crave.

I climb into bed willing him to come to me, I need to have that final conversation. He hadn't left a note. I think suicide notes were invented by Hollywood. They're mainly a myth, I later learn. Yet I am so desperate for that bit of understanding about what has happened.

But Joe doesn't appear in a vision at the bottom of my bed. He provides no answers.

I start talking out loud, hoping – somewhere – he can hear me.

I shout at the air, raging. 'YOU FUCKING CUNT!'

Monday, August 10:
Telling the world

For weeks I'd wake up every morning and talk to Joe with that kind of bitter fury. Hatred, almost. 'Don't speak ill of the dead,' people traditionally say.

Fuck that. I had so much hurt and anger that negative obscenities were virtually all that came out my mouth for a while. All directed at the mate I missed and loved.

When I was on my own I cried and I cried.

I took three days off work in the aftermath. I've no idea now how I really filled that time. But on the Monday, I knew we owed the Capital listeners an explanation for why we came off air so suddenly – and why we hadn't come back to work.

My executive producer and I wrote some words together. And everyone squeezed into the studio to hear me read them out. I steeled myself to do it, and there were tears along the way.

Here's an edited version of what I told to the listeners that day:

'We're back after what was a really, massive sudden break on our show. And we wanted to just be able to take a minute to explain a little bit more about why we went off air last week.

Here on Capital Breakfast we are a massive family. We've got

SHARING SAVES LIVES

all of our team in the studio right now. And you as well. You're part of our family – you listen every single morning, you're part of that.

And we wanted to share with you – there's no other way of saying it – some really sad news.

I never thought I'd have to do this, ever.

Last Tuesday, very suddenly, we lost one of our best friends.

My best friend and our colleague, producer Joe.

Everybody who works at Capital was completely devastated and we were trying to process this all together, and we were all around each other.

We wanted to be able to share this news with you as well, so that you just understand a little bit more about where we're coming from.

Joe has worked for Global, the parent company, for nine years. He was the first person I met when I walked in the door and I remember thinking, 'Who's this guy? He's a bit of a Del Boy'.

He's worked at LBC before, he was with me right from my very first show, he taught me everything. I don't know sitting in a radio studio without him.

It is really, really weird.

Every huge A-lister that you ever hear on this show? They know who he is. Everyone.

He's the person that they spoke with first and if you've ever called into this show… he was the person that picked up the phone. He's always been playing the games as well with us. He's the person that I'd sit here and rinse constantly.

He's the person we share our mornings with every day. And Sian and Sonny, and our exceptional team of producers who keep the show moving.

We wanted to be able to tell you a little bit about producer Joe as a person.

He really couldn't do enough for people.

He was the nicest guy that I know.

Hands down. He was kind and caring.

He really loved dogs. He was obsessed with his daily step count.

He never ironed his clothes

He loved his family. So much. His dad Ivan. His mum Celia and sister Lou.

He loved his friends.

The thing that he loved most of all was doing this show and he loved you listening right now and he loved making you happy.

There are so many things that you would have heard on Capital that were him.

He was like a genius just coming up with these ideas. And it was driven by the reaction from you every day.

He was playful, silly and our best mate.

This person is someone who is my absolute brother.

Joe, you're gonna be so missed by us here at Capital every single day.

You loved coming in and entertaining people every morning, singing so horrendously out of key, and we're going to carry on making people laugh for you. And because of that, we know the show's gotta go on. So thank you so much, Joe. We love you so much.'

I managed to somehow get to the end, hot tears streaming down my red cheeks, and we played a clip of Joe's funniest moments.

Going back to work without him felt like returning to a

place of trauma. I felt like I was the town widow, whose husband everyone knew and loved. People were uncomfortable, tiptoeing around me and didn't know what to say to me.

His jacket was still hanging up in the corner. Yet no one was sitting in his seat.

October 2020:
Why? Why? Why?

I desperately, desperately wanted my mate back. Just to hear his voice. And trying to make sense of his sudden absence, while going through the normal routine, was very strange.

I frequently felt a huge hatred for Joe some days.

And I also had this massive guilt, about not being there to stop him. My thoughts went down a warren hole of negativity. Had I been the cause of this?

If I hadn't had my success, would Joe still be alive? That was my train of thought.

I was terrified by thinking that I was like the puppet, the famous one. But Joe was the puppeteer, the clever, talented one making it all happen behind the scenes. Joe was in the wings, watching me get bigger and earn more money and seeing me buy my own flat.

I couldn't help wondering… if I hadn't done this well, would Joe still be alive and still be with his family now?

I know he didn't really resent me. It probably wasn't rational. But these were the dark thoughts I really worried about late into the night. Had I caused this? Had I done this to someone so important in my life, who I loved so much?

Any bereavement counsellor will tell you that there are many stages of grief – denial, anger, guilt, bargaining, acceptance –

but they don't come in the same order for everyone. And you can go round and round the cycle, again and again.

When you've lost someone you love to suicide, it's complex.

I became obsessed. Why? Why? Why?

When the idea was floated about making a documentary on suicide in the October after Joe's death, I immediately wanted in. My management were contacted by the BBC. And after respectfully seeking the permission of Joe's family, I said yes.

Some people thought I was mad, that it was too soon. But I'd become grimly preoccupied with the shocking statistics surrounding suicide and young males. I knew from a purely selfish point of view that if I signed up to do a TV show, I'd have access to speaking to all of the top experts. I needed to understand more.

I was driven by this strong urge for other people to sit up and pay attention to this almost 'silent emergency' that was happening in Britain – and that's exactly what we ended up calling the documentary.

We made this against the backdrop of the second lockdown. I was very raw. But I wanted to be brutally honest about my own experiences, even though I worried people would think, 'Who's this privileged celebrity kid thinking he is? What does he know?'

My dad was fully supportive of me making the show. Mum, however, was a bit concerned about my mental health. She was worried it would send me into a spiral. Or at the very least might signal the end of my career.

I didn't want it to be all 'woe is me, I've lost my mate'.

But I really felt it was my duty, as Joe's best mate, to do the research, put in the work, and use the platform I had to spread this message.

SHARING SAVES LIVES

When it was announced we were making the documentary, I got a lot of abuse online, saying someone with my privilege had no right to be talking about suicide or mental health. They said it was nepotism, that I had any platform, and that it was more nepotism because it was the broadcaster Anneka Rice's son, Josh Allott, who was the director!

I didn't give a fuck about the criticism, I wasn't really thinking straight. I was so determined that if I could make just one person think twice before taking their own life, it would be worth it.

For five months at weekends, the director Josh and I went to meet different experts, loved ones whose lives had been affected by suicide, and young people who were struggling with their mental health. It really hit home how bad young men are about talking about their feelings. As a society we have all been conditioned that men shouldn't cry, or express their emotions, we were supposed to simply 'man up' – and shut up.

But the more I learned, the more I saw how that had to change. Young kids deserve more than this.

It wasn't easy, there was so much I didn't know. And I was very shy about promoting the show, with all the privileges I have. Yet it felt the only useful thing to be doing in the circumstances.

Since I've made the documentary I've become part of a whole community of people affected by suicide. Something I could never have predicted or ever wanted.

PART 2.

IT'S ALL IN YOUR HEAD

The Big List Of My Life

ROMAN KEMP – ARE YOU REALLY OK?

Since the shock of Joe's death, I've realised that everything in life has potential to affect your mental health.

So, for the purposes of this book, I sat down one day and made a list of everything that matters to me, the experiences that shaped who I am, and the things that happen in my life that affect how I'm feeling.

We all have our own narratives, but I found that coming up with this list gave me a better and deeper understanding of myself. And having that curiosity about my own inner landscape and mental health can help me see it more clearly.

So I'll talk to you honestly and openly about how it's shaped me to become the person I am today...

THE BIG LIST OF MY LIFE

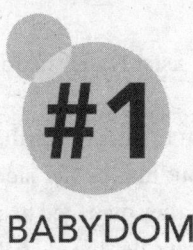

BABYDOM

***'If someone asks me what's the best thing
to ever happen to me is, it's the parents
I was given'***

I haven't always been someone who has struggled with their mental health, honestly!

I'll rewind a bit to some happier tales. And I was a very jolly little chap as a kid.

Mum says that I came out during my birth Superman-style, with my raised arm above my head. Later, a psychic told her that when a baby is born in this superhero position (which frankly sounds pretty painful for my mum) it means your child is 'ready to receive'. Ready to receive what exactly? I've never had the faintest idea!

But Mum and Dad were into being pretty alternative at that time, so they probably thought it had great significance on the kind of character I was going to be in later life.

Dad was working on a film in Los Angeles at the time Mum was expecting me. His band, Spandau Ballet, had split up by then, and Dad was busy carving out a successful acting career for himself.

Officially, women over 36 weeks pregnant aren't supposed to fly anywhere. No flight attendant wants to be dealing with a woman in labour, do they? So I should have been born in

London, where my big sister Harley had arrived, two-and-a-half years earlier.

But Dad didn't want to miss the birth, and Mum didn't want to go through it without him by her side, so despite her being nine months pregnant, they managed to use strategically-placed coats and bags to smuggle her big old belly through the airport in England – and onto a transatlantic flight.

However, almost as soon as they landed in California, Mum started having contractions… little me had decided it was time to make my grand entrance into the world and bag myself a dual American-British passport… thanks very much guys! (If you've ever seen me play football on Soccer Aid over the years, and wondered why I play for the Rest of the World team, this is the reason why.)

So with Mum in the full grips of labour, and Dad in sheer panic, they madly dashed to get to the Cedars-Sinai Hospital – just in time for my dramatic arrival.

All sorts of celebrities – from Madonna and Patrick Swayze to Elizabeth Taylor and Frank Sinatra – have been patients at the Cedars-Sinai over the years. Beyonce gave birth here, as did many of the Kardashians.

So, I like to think of myself as a bit of a trend-setter!

Mum always has this belief that the first decision you make in life is picking who your parents are (I did warn you she can be a bit 'woo woo', my mum). But I prefer to imagine it's like in the Keanu Reeves film The Matrix, where everyone is in their little pods and you get assigned someone, and that's where you end up.

Who knows how life works, but if someone asks me what's the best thing to ever happen to me, it's undoubtedly the parents I was given. Not because they're famous, and certainly not

THE BIG LIST OF MY LIFE

because they're rich – they've endured real financial struggles over the years – but quite simply because they're the world's nicest people. Everyone says that about my dad Martin and mum Shirlie – they're nice.

Even I can admit that I wasn't an ugly baby and if the home videos are anything to go by, Harley – then a toddler – struggled when I was born. It didn't seem like she was keen on sharing the limelight or our parents' affections with little old me.

I was a chunky little thing with big blue eyes, long lashes and a mop of blond hair. I totally looked like a little girl, so that's exactly how Mum styled me, posing me up for many pictures bizarrely lying naked in flower beds half the time. Cheers, Mum!

Because it was super hot in LA, and Mum and Dad were hippy-ish, I was left naked a lot and stuck out in the sun. Apparently, it was so I could soak up vitamin D.

One of Dad's favourite ways to rinse me is re-telling the time when I was just a week old and they'd plopped me out in the garden. There I was, butt naked on a rug, when a huge, hovering bumblebee buzzed right in for the kill…. stinging me directly on my delicate newborn penis.

OUCH!

Funnily enough, I wailed a lot.

And to this day I still blame that bumblebee for stunting my growth down there…

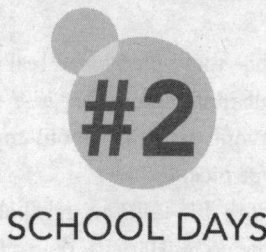

SCHOOL DAYS

'Roman won't stop talking...'

Dad now admits that when I was growing up he sometimes worried about me because I was such a little entertainer, I'd be in the middle of the floor in my element holding court, and loving every minute of it.

Yet he recognised there was probably a flip side to this happy extrovert kid – he instinctively felt like with all those massive 'ups' I revelled in, running around on top of the world, there inevitably had to be some 'downs' too. And of course, he turned out to be right.

Though to be honest, those low moments didn't really start manifesting themselves until I hit my teens.

We moved back to England when I was three. And I was enrolled in a local prep school near where we lived in north London.

I really struggled concentrating on books as a kid, I just got easily distracted. Mind like a butterfly. I'm still like that now. I'm not a reader. I will pick up a book, and by the time I've got to the end of chapter one, I can have entirely forgotten what it's about. People at work can't believe I'm real because I can read an autocue word-perfectly, and then somehow not really take in a single word of what I've just said.

I was definitely what you'd call a high-energy kid, bouncing off the walls, seeking attention and showing off. I can still be like that now. I've often wondered whether I have a mild form of ADHD, though I've never been officially diagnosed with anything. My teachers did all reckon I had dyscalculia, because I was always so, so bad with numbers. Dyscalculia is a bit like dyslexia, but instead of struggling with reading words and letters, it was always maths and arithmetic that I just couldn't get my head around.

So I was always very average academically. School reports always said the same thing: 'Roman won't concentrate, Roman can't sit still, Roman won't stop talking.'

At parents' evenings lots of the female teachers seemed to get quite excited and make a little bit of extra effort with their appearance, perhaps hoping my dad might come along to the appointments. He never did though. It was always Mum who did the school stuff.

He'd landed the role of villainous club owner Steve Owen in EastEnders when I was five, and was on the show for nearly four years, just when it was getting huge ratings in the days when there were far fewer channels to choose from. He was in some massive storylines, including the murder of his love interest Saskia, after he buried an ashtray into her skull (as you do).

One time, when I was about six, a fire engine came to school and all the firemen turned up in their cool uniforms to show us the truck and all the equipment and teach us about fire safety. It was the stuff of every little boy's fantasy. Yet clearly I felt my nose was put out of joint by how impressed all my classmates were by the fire guys.

At the end of their demo, when they asked all the kids if they had any questions, I proudly stuck my hand up. 'You may think that's cool,' I announced to all gathered. 'But my dad is

Steve Owen!' I'm sure it was desperately cringe-worthy for everyone to witness – but I've always had zero filter and don't get embarrassed. Sometimes to my detriment.

At weekends and in the summer time I played football at Alexandra Palace, or Ally Pally as locals call it.

Mum came to pick me up after summer school one afternoon and found me – aged just five or six – standing on top of a table and giving all these much older teenagers and adult coaches quite a show.

I was belting out a full rendition of the 1970s Donna Summer hit Hot Stuff, but it was the Arsenal team version, with all the words changed to being about Arsenal players. I knew every lyric and hip thrust and was really going for it with not the slightest bit of shame. My confidence could be insane back then, I loved performing and from the home videos I reckon I was pretty good at it.

While I loved the chance to show off at school, knuckling down and actually working was never my forte.

Dad was the more strict parent when it came to working. He was always the one who said, 'You've got to do your homework, Ro.' Mum however was a much easier touch. She knew what I was like.

Mum and Dad's parenting style was definitely what you'd call 'bohemian'. They always made a point of treating Harley and I as their mates, rather than their children to boss around. It definitely caused some controversy at the time, not everyone approved of their laid-back attitude. But as kids we always felt respected and heard.

Growing up, Harley and I had few rules to stick to. I don't remember ever being told what we could or couldn't do or could and couldn't watch on TV. There were no bans on screen time, and we never heard the words, 'You're too young to be watching that.'

In fact, I remember one of the first films I ever watched with my dad, when I must have been six, was The Texas Chainsaw Massacre. Many parents would be horrified by this – the disturbing American classic from the '70s had been banned in several countries! But I think Dad wanted me to understand how horror movies work, he wanted me to know that CGI is not real, and he'd patiently explain how every scene was made and what this person or that one was doing at the time, to make it realistic on screen.

####

'Coming over to our house was like getting a crash course in learning to be an adult. And my parents adored having the house full of youngsters'

####

And if something upset me or gave me nightmares, Mum and Dad would just shrug, 'Well, if you're going to watch it and be scared, that's your call, don't watch it if it's scaring you.'

We were really given incredible amounts of freedom.

So when Grand Theft Auto came out and was massively popular, I was probably the only kid I knew who was actually allowed to play it. Funnily enough, many of my young friends' parents thought a violent video game about nicking cars probably wasn't suitable for primary school-age kids to be playing!

I'd have friends come over and they'd think it was great I was allowed to do so much. In fact, they'd often specifically ask, 'Can I come over to your house so I can watch South Park or play GTA?' (South Park was another rather 'adult' cartoon which we loved.)

There were some kids whose mums and dads specifically didn't allow them to come and play at our house because we were apparently allowed to do as we pleased.

But the kids who did come, they'd love it! Coming over to our house was like getting a crash course in learning to be an adult. And my parents adored having the house full of youngsters and made real efforts to have proper chats with us all.

It wasn't like Mum and Dad didn't impose any rules. We weren't feral. They still wanted to instil in us important values and teach us that if we wanted to do more 'grown-up' things, then we had to know how to behave properly too.

When Mum and Dad had friends over, we were encouraged to sit at the table with the adults and take a proper part in the conversation. It was the opposite of the Victorian 'be seen but not heard' approach towards children.

They wanted us to take an active part in listening to different opinions and being able to hold conversations. They taught us that everyone has a right to their own opinion and while you don't have to always agree with it, you need to respect it. That's such an important life lesson and certainly helps me in my job now, as I absolutely love meeting new people and listening to their point of view.

People might assume our house would have been filled with famous people when I was growing up. But it wasn't like that at all. In reality, Mum and Dad are quite homely people, they're insanely loved-up, even after nearly 40 years together, and are very happy just being in their own company. Not hosting famous types. They didn't throw parties, they're just not extravagant people like that.

We're such a close-knit unit of four. Christmas in our house was magical, and yes I fully recognise I was a spoiled kid because I'd get so many presents – a bike, video games, the latest Batman toy.

But as well as the stockings and presents under the tree, in our house we also had this slightly more unusual tradition – which probably sounds weird to everyone else – of pulling down all the blinds, locking the doors and literally cocooning ourselves inside. Then we'd spend most of the day eating and laughing, and watching all the Christmas telly together.

The four of us have always been insanely close. And that unit has always been my absolute bedrock.

TEENAGE KICKS

'When I learned people were judging me...'

From 13 onwards, that's when life gets real, isn't it? You stop being a little kid and the responsibilities of life seem to kick in a bit. These were the years when Mum first noticed I started suffering with poor mental health. But it crept up on me slowly, probably as my hormones started changing.

When you hit adolescence is when you start comparing yourself to your peers at this age, isn't it? Am I tall enough? Am I athletic enough? And that classic pubescent concern... who'll be the first one to get pubic hair? Man, did I feel proud when those babies started sprouting!

I'd say I was pretty average in all these areas. I grew taller than some of my mates, (I'm 6ft 2in now). And while I was never the most athletic team member, I wasn't bad either. And I could play football. Football has always been my passion, as I'll describe later.

But I was basically a real middle-of-the-road kind of teenager which, let's face it, is a nice place to be. No one wants to stand out for the wrong reasons at that age.

After we'd moved out to Hertfordshire, to be closer to the EastEnders studio, I'd attended a prep school, York House, followed by an all-boys public school in Berkhamsted. That meant getting up at 5am every day to catch the 5.30am bus from our house in Rickmansworth all the way out to Berkie. Good preparation, I guess, for all the early starts I do now.

Berkhamsted School was a smart, fee-paying place, opened by Henry VIII no less. I wanted to go there because a few of my mates from prep school were too, including one of my best mates, Charlie. Plus my parents thought it suited me as the drama department was supposed to be good there. Clearly, I was never going to be a great academic scholar, and seemed more likely to end up on stage.

I was nervous on my first day. Happy to be out of my bright purple blazer I'd worn at prep school, I felt all grown-up and well, upper-class in my suit and tie.

And because the school was right in the middle of the town it felt much more adult. The school drummed it into us from the beginning that we had a responsibility to behave well and not piss around as we were 'representing the establishment' each time we walked around from lesson A on one side of town, to lesson B on the other side.

One thing I really appreciate now is that we were all encouraged to have our own voice. It was certainly an institution that bred confident young men who were given the space to be creative. Many of my year group are now in the public eye and are super successful. You might have heard of them:

- Olajide Olayinka Williams – better known as KSI. He's one of the biggest YouTubers on the planet, and part of the massively successful Sidemen.

- Simon Minter – goes under the name Miniminter, another huge YouTube personality and member of the Sidemen.

- Jonathan Bond – he's the goalkeeper for LA Galaxy.

- Alexander Kotz – professionally he works as Elderbrook, is doing great as a musician, songwriter and producer.

- Alice Liveing (the sixth form at school was co-ed) – a personal trainer who is doing brilliantly with a Primark campaign and educating the masses on all things health and fitness.

Mainly, I felt grateful that I was fortunate enough to be at a place where there was no expectation that I ever had to go to university. There wasn't that pressure.

Everyone assumed because of who my dad was I would end up acting, it was like even from the beginning my future destiny was all mapped out for me.

And I didn't really question it at the time. I happily accepted that was my fate.

So I never worried about what I would do for a career because everyone else seemed to assume it would come naturally to me. I thought, 'I don't have to listen to these lessons, I know what I'm going to do with my life, I'll be OK.'

That gave me comfort and confidence at the time, but perhaps in hindsight wasn't the best thing when it came to getting qualifications and passing exams...

I winged my whole way through that school.

One thing I began not enjoying, however, was becoming well aware by these teenage years that people were judging me on who my parents were. Or that's how I felt at least.

'Think you're special?' kids might sneer. Or sing Spandau songs or make EastEnders ashtray jokes at me. I developed a bit of a tough exterior, so if someone threw an insult at me, about my dad, or my mum, or my so-called celebrity privilege, I became the master of hitting them straight back with a joke. Or sometimes, I'd get in there first, sending myself up before they could even say anything. I was developing a comedy defence mechanism. It was mainly just teenage boys doing what they do really, but with what I'd describe as a bit of a mean edge.

If it wasn't spiky banter, it seemed like the opposite could also be true – that other kids only wanted to be my friend because of who my folks were. It did make me a bit wary of people. And that's been carried with me later in life. I think I've become quite good at reading the people who are genuine. I'm a bit like my mum, though, we both tend to size people up before we trust them. Harley and Dad are much more open and quicker to give others the benefit of the doubt.

Another thing I definitely inherited from Mum was our ability to worry. Mum is a natural-born worrier. She worries about everything! If I chat to her on the phone and I'm walking at the same time, she'll be on the other end reminding me to look both ways as I'm crossing the road. Mum – I'm 29!!

As a teen, anxieties about Mum and Dad's marriage started creeping in. Not because they ever seemed likely to split up. Far from it. But because I loved them SO MUCH and wanted them to stay happy forever in our little unit I started fearing they'd separate and life would change. I guess around that age I had friends whose parents were divorcing and I was terrified mine could do the same.

Mum actually took me to a therapist for a couple of sessions where we talked this through, and they helped me try and cut out some of these anxieties. It did make a difference, and made me more open to therapy in the future, which I'm grateful for.

When I was 15, Dad reunited with Spandau Ballet in 2009 for a world tour, and he was back in the newspapers again. That was cool and exciting, and yet and as result, I also felt a bit more… visible, somehow.

But if I felt like I got a harder time from the other kids because of this, I also know I got a much easier ride from my teachers because of who my dad was. I got away with a lot more in terms of not working and dressing however I wanted to.

By your teens you're fully aware of who's cool and who's not. And I really wanted to be cool. I started expressing myself with how I looked, pushing the boundaries of the school's strict dress code.

When I needed new school trousers Mum took me to British Home Stores.

'Mum, we need to be shopping in the girls section,' I insisted.

'Here we go,' she probably thought, wondering if I was going to tell her I was actually transgender. Not that Mum would have batted an eyelid about that, to be honest. Her and Dad are nothing if not open minded.

But no, I explained that I wanted to shop in the girls' section just because I had my heart set on having Very Tight Trousers. Skinny jeans were the fashion – and I badly wanted in on the action.

My mates constantly tell me my fashion is horrendous. Looking back at the photos – I can see why.

But Mum was happy to indulge me and let me dress how I damn well pleased, so she dutifully bought me the skinny-legged girls trousers I wanted in BHS. Happy days.

The school rule was that we were expected to wear our hair in a classic short back and sides, with no hair allowed anywhere on your face.

But somehow for years I got away with an asymmetrical haircut. I'd shaved one side of my hair and then wore the other side completely flopped down my face, emo style, covering my entire eye and cheek.

It felt like a competition to see how far your fringe could come down and naturally, I wanted to win it. I spent hours on the school bus straightening my hair every day. I kept my trusty pair of GHD straighteners in my school bag, and they came everywhere with me.

I also went through a stage of bleaching the fringe blond, and at one point I had a David Beckham-style mohawk (I got Mum to frost the tips like he had) and I even sported a mullet at one point, again inspired by a footballer.

I was the only kid at school who got away with it, which must have really pissed off the other kids in hindsight. Others pupils would be packed off into town with a fiver to get a regular cut at the barber's. Yet I think the teachers all accepted it from me because they had us labelled as the 'artistic, quirky family'.

One time it was brought up by a teacher, and good old Mum sent in a letter saying, 'This is Roman's way of expressing himself.' They probably thought I was a right dick, but I never got asked about my 'interesting' hair choices again.

Mum would happily take me to Selco, in Camden, which is like a builders' warehouse, so I could go and get myself dubious fashion items, like a toilet chain which I'd then tie around my trousers. I imagine I looked a right state, but if I was 'expressing myself' through my style choices, then Mum and Dad were always happy.

They found their own styles in the '80s, you only need to look at old photos to see how unintentionally hilarious they looked half the time (sorry folks). But they always argue that back then clothes were still an important and creative opportunity to express yourself. They mourn those good old days now.

They were probably less happy about the fact that I was so bad at maths. Despite paying for me to have a tutor on the side for two years, when it came to my GCSE maths I turned up to the exam, wrote my name on the paper, then got up and left. Unsurprisingly, I came away with just a 'U' in that subject.

Because I was in the bottom set for so many subjects, I often played up for attention. I became the class clown. The joker.

####

> **'Dad literally unleashed hell on me when he heard. 'You can never, ever be part of anything like that again, Ro,' he warned me sternly'**

####

I had a brilliant art teacher, Mr Thomas, and sometimes he'd let me off doing any work at all if I stood up in front of the class and did a full performance or impression of another teacher. It sounds quite strange and unconventional, but I owe a lot to teachers like that who just allowed me to be myself.

I was granted more freedom than most of my peers, and as a teen I'd get the Tube to Camden Market most weekends, where I'd normally get a band T-shirt or new hoodie. The one place that I wasn't allowed to go to was Brixton, which is ironic as that's exactly where I ended up getting my first place.

We got up to a few things I never told my parents about. Like shoplifting.

I'm not proud of that, but we would dare each other to take small things like trinkets or lighters – little teenage trophies, I guess. It was about the thrill of being caught. And if we did get caught, which happened several times, I'd be the first person to quickly front the situation up, apologise, and somehow talk my way out of it.

When I was 14 we were followed by these older lads one time. I had my phone in the inside pocket and I knew I was being followed. I had this sharp thing pointed in my back, and I heard a gruff voice behind me telling me to hand over my wallet and phone. He took my wallet, there was probably only a fiver in there. But I didn't tell him I had my phone. I kept it hidden, which was totally dumb.

Mum and Dad always lectured me that if ever I got mugged or asked to hand over my phone, I should immediately do that. It's not worth being stabbed over your phone.

I got home and didn't admit what had happened. I think I found that thrill of being in danger was exciting though. It was the first but not the last time I got mugged.

I suppose I was very lucky never to get into any real trouble.

The only time Dad has ever pulled me aside to really have words with me was when I got into a few scrapes with other lads.

I got into a couple of fights at school, and then later in my early 20s I was once in a bit of a bar brawl. It wasn't particularly messy, a few punches, some name calling, that type of thing. I think that's one of the only times I remember Dad coming down on me really hard and having a proper go at me.

I'd been recognised and singled out because of who I was, or who Dad was more accurately, and while I'm not a fighter by nature I did fight back that time and came home with a few cuts on my hands and stuff. Dad literally unleashed hell on me when he heard. 'You can never, ever be part of anything like that again, Ro,' he warned me sternly. 'You have to understand that your reputation is at stake, you make one silly mistake like that and it's all over.'

'But he hit me first!' I protested. Dad didn't care. He warned me that those situations were things I just had to walk away from and couldn't get involved with. He was absolutely right though and I've listened to him. I've since been in scenarios where people have yelled hideous things at me, trying to wind me up saying stuff about my parents or something I've said, and I've learned to just walk away.

People have tweeted me in the past saying, 'I hope you die in a pool of your own AIDS.' Just stupid, horrible stuff, but it's part of the job and you just have to accept there are some times when you just can't retaliate.

It was an important lesson Dad taught me and one I've had to adhere to ever since.

THE BIG LIST OF MY LIFE

DAD

'He's not scared to show his emotions, he's taught me that real men do cry'

Anyone who's seen us together on telly will know that Dad and I rinse each other constantly. Whether it's on Celebrity Gogglebox or Weekend Best, how we banter and take the piss out of each other on telly is exactly what we're like in real life.

But underneath the jokes, Dad is my hero and my best mate and we are insanely close. I am absolutely blessed that we have one of the best father-and-son relationships of anyone I know.

We can and do talk about anything and everything. Dad will cheerfully tell me – and all the viewers at home – about his daily 'manscaping' preferences. He likes to sit on the loo backwards so he can shave his bits and handily use the top of the cistern to rest the razor on. (Er, thanks for that tip Dad, much appreciated.) And once I had actually to walk off the sofa during Gogglebox when Dad insisted that I would have found Mum 'tasty' when she was younger. (Ewwww. That made me feel quite ill thinking about that.)

But from when I was born until I went to school, my main memories of Dad are of him being really very poorly. Growing up, I was used to seeing Dad with no hair, and feeling sick a lot.

It wasn't frightening to me because I simply didn't know any different.

Dad had led a seemingly charmed life – huge success in the band, then meeting my mum, the love of his life, and having two kids he adored. But his world turned upside down in 1995 when it was discovered he had a brain tumour, the size of a crushed grapefruit, at the back of his head.

Luckily, it was benign and on the outside of his brain. It took two to three years to get rid of. Then, just as they were about to give Dad the all-clear, he was dealt a second blow – the doctors realised there was another large tumour, this time growing from the inside of his brain. It was also benign, but the second growth was more dangerous and complex to treat because of where it was positioned.

And for a year or so of his life, he seriously thought he was dying because surgery didn't seem an option. He was only in his mid-30s, with two young kids and a wife to support. All the money he'd made from Spandau Ballet's success had been spent on medical bills in the States, where he needed to be treated.

In the end, after nearly two years of analysis, doctors were finally able to reduce it using an early form of Gamma Knife technology. His career was totally derailed for a while. But, thank God, he's fine now.

He must have been absolutely terrified. I don't know how he and Mum got through that really.

I was just a toddler at the time, so had no real understanding of what he was going through. Mum did such a fantastic job of protecting Harley and me from how serious the situation was. Despite her worrying nature, when the shit hit the fan Mum became a real warrior.

Dad spent most of his time back then in a room in the front

of the house, which was his office. He would be in there looking very frail and bald. His body was covered in a mass of scars from various tubes and from when things got messed up during surgery. Those scars are insane.

Until I was about six I thought all these vivid red lines marking his skin were from a shark attack, because that's what he always told me. So of course I believed him, and that's what I told all the kids at school.

But the tumours left other problems behind. Dad became epileptic, dependent on medication – he was on morphine for eight weeks – and he became so dyslexic he couldn't even read a script. He still struggles now. He had to teach himself how to talk again and how to walk again.

For a good-looking dude, who had enjoyed all that success in the band, and then had managed to make the leap into acting – with an amazing turn in The Krays – it must have come as a completely shocking headfuck.

Yet we were never made to tiptoe around him, and he never shut the door on us, we just got used to Dad being Dad, in his room.

However shit he must have felt at times, he was never self-pitying, and he always put us first. One of my favourite memories is the time I proudly took him in a picture I'd drawn of Batman dressed as a cowboy, like Woody from Toy Story. I'm sure it was awful, yet Dad was always so encouraging about everything I did, and made a huge fuss.

'It's fantastic, Ro!' he praised. 'The best Batman cowboy I've ever seen!'

Dad then went to his fax machine (remember those?) and told me he was sending it somewhere very special. I was totally in awe, did my Dad really have a hotline to a superhero?

Obviously it was going nowhere apart from the front room but, sure enough, three days later Dad announced that he had a special gift for me – and presented me with an Adam West-signed picture of Batman. It was the very best thing I could have imagined.

Dad would always go out of his way to make us feel special and loved like that, and play along with all the imaginative games you loved as a kid.

At Christmas he'd go all out to make Santa Claus real, traipsing flour footprints all over the floor. I think we stopped believing the year we found the flour on Dad's own shoe but we played along for many more years to make sure we kept getting all the presents under the tree. And I never told Dad that I'd always been a bit scared of Father Christmas, I didn't like the idea of this old man being in our house so I'd make Harley go and check he'd gone before I came downstairs.

Dad started writing a book and he'd be there in his room tapping away on one of those very first Apple Mac computers. I didn't know it at the time, but he'd first started writing his autobiography, True, for me and Harley because he genuinely thought he was dying, and he wanted to write down everything about his life for us to read his story so we would really know him when he was gone.

When I was old enough, I was allowed to read it, and every so often I'll still pick it up and go back and read bits again.

It wasn't until I started talking about my own mental health publicly, that I had my first adult discussion with Dad about his. After the tumour, and while grappling with the effects it had had on him, he admitted that for three years he felt like he was in his own little, isolated bubble.

Many men of his generation didn't share things – like talking about their feelings – with their mates. Or indeed anyone else. They just bottled everything up.

It was Mum who realised he needed some help, she could see how lost he was, and in the end she slightly tricked him into seeing someone to talk about it all. She packed him off to a cranial osteopath who was also a trained therapist, and he got him to open up as he worked on his back.

Like many people I guess, Dad was comfortable receiving help for a physical ailment but would have brushed off the thought of seeing a talking therapist as something 'other people' did. He grew up off the Essex Road and had a very humble background before he hit the big time. Therapy wasn't on his agenda.

Dad had never experienced depression until the years when he was recovering from having the brain tumour removed. Now, he admits it left him on the floor – as if the world was happening outside of his own bubble and he couldn't get back into it.

Talking to the therapist for those weeks meant he could finally get it all out. He told me that he cried his eyes out every day for a while, which gradually released all his pent-up emotions, and enabled him to come back out of his bubble and feel part of the world again. It helped him to clear the fog and he could live his life again.

When I chat with Dad now, which I do all the time because we're so close, we never mention his tumours. Not because he's embarrassed or because he doesn't want me to worry, but just because he's accepted what happened to him, he's happy with his lot, and he's moved on.

His view is very much that you have to stand up and deal with what you've been given in life. There are times when you don't enjoy life, for a couple of weeks, or a couple of months, or even a couple of years. But it's how you bounce back from that. Are you going to be someone who is a victim, and blames things for how you are, or are you going to recognise it as a moment in life and it's something you can use to build your character?

That's Dad's mentality. As he acknowledges, when other people look at our family they're going to think we've had it good, we've got nothing to complain about. He's spot-on. And that's a really valuable life lesson he instilled.

Dad is not one to lecture me about any of this stuff, these are things I've learned by watching his example.

The first thing I ever saw him in was The Krays, the film about notorious gangsters Reggie and Ronnie. I've watched Dad die on screen several times. I've seen him blown up, had his head squashed, I've seen him overdose on drugs.

It's been strange, almost comical seeing Dad play all these villains over the years because in real life he's the most gentle, caring and sensitive man you could imagine.

One of the most important lessons Dad has ingrained in me is to always have respect for other people. If you've made someone feel like shit in an argument, you apologise for that, even if you don't agree with them. He always tries to understand the other person's point of view.

At 60, Dad still has his fair share of female admirers, which he's a bit sheepish about and which Mum thinks is hilarious and ridiculous. But I have to admit he's the best-looking member of our family and in some ways I'm quite looking forward to going grey like him one day, he's working the old silver fox look so well.

People always ask if it was hard growing up under his shadow. But the truth is, Dad is my hero and I'm too proud of him to feel anything coming close to resentment or jealousy. The only times we get competitive is when we're playing FIFA (which, can I just say, I smash him at). Dad has shown me unconditional love and been a constant cheerleader throughout my life. He's been a fantastic role model for my own mental health because he's not scared to show his emotions, he's taught me that real men do cry. And when he needed to speak to a therapist for his post-illness depression, he learned how opening up really can work, which has encouraged me to do the same.

Three random things you might not know about my dad:

- Dad is a very clean guy, he likes everything to be tidy and cleared up immediately. He's almost a little bit OCD, I'd say. Every Christmas or birthday celebration, Dad would stand there with a big bin-liner waiting to collect the wrapping paper. He literally cannot stand the mess. I'm sure I've lost hundreds of pounds' worth of gift vouchers over the years by Dad helpfully 'recycling them'.

- Dad is the kind of guy who is happy to walk around at home naked. He lets it hang out with no embarrassment. I've got used to it, but I've lost count of the times a girlfriend has come over and gone, 'Oh my God – I've just seen your dad's arse!'

- When Dad performed at Live Aid in 1985 (two billion viewers no less!) he was flown in a helicopter to Wembley Stadium, and thought it was a wind-up when he discovered Noel Edmonds in the cockpit. Who knew Noel was a licensed helicopter pilot?

#5 MUM

'She was the person who first recognised my depression, and the person who saved my life...'

Being the son of Martin Kemp means people often come up to me in the street, in cafés, wherever I am, and say, 'I love your dad! He's so amazing!' Blah blah blah.

It's nice that people like my dad, and nice they want to talk about him, don't get me wrong. But I always want to say to them, 'And what about my mum?' Because my mum is wicked.

I always want to stand up and sing her praises – she played at Live Aid too, she had a number one record, she was part of the first Western pop band to ever play live in China, you know what I mean?

Mum is one of the toughest people you will meet. She left school with no qualifications, but she's one of the most capable humans I know. And a little bit bossy...

She grew up one of four siblings in a tiny council house, sharing a bed tucked up between her two sisters. She adored her mum – my nan – but her dad was not a nice man. Their constant fighting and screaming gave her bad anxiety. It was shit for her, but what it did for me was wonderful, because it made her determined to raise her own family in a loving and calm environment.

When Dad was very sick, it was Mum who held all the shit

together. Not only was she terrified of losing him to the brain tumour, she had to keep the show on the road with me and Harley, protecting us and giving us a happy, carefree childhood. And that she really did.

I didn't realise until much later that she went through bankruptcy in the aftermath of Dad's illness. All I remember at the time was that we moved to a smaller house, then we lost the nice Jeep we had, and were suddenly driving around in a much smaller car. Holidays might have become less bougie, but we had love in huge quantities. I have nothing to complain about – I was never kept awake worrying about any of this, because Mum did everything possible to make sure our lives were unaffected.

Since then, I've asked her, 'Mum, how did you deal with all that? How the hell did you cope?' Did she think about planning his funeral? Was she terrified about being a widow and raising two kids with no money?

And Mum just says that she couldn't think like that. She likened it to drowning, where the only thing you can do in that moment is fight to keep your head above water. The survival instinct kicks in. She didn't think too far ahead to the future or the 'what ifs'. She just lived day by day.

Which might be a good lesson for many of us.

I never went without anything I needed, there were always Christmas and birthday presents and the fees were paid so I could go to football training each week at Ally Pally, which was such a large part of my life as a kid.

Mum is always looking for the next reason to be positive.

Never once has Mum taken the tough love approach with me, she's simply been there as a constant source of nurture, love and care throughout all my ups and downs. Protecting me like a tigress.

The first time I really realised she had my back, and was like a mate, not just a mum, was when I was eight.

I hadn't done my school homework one time, there was probably a family dinner or something going on, so my lovely mum sent me in with a letter for the teacher apologising and explaining why it hadn't been done and that it wasn't my fault.

When I handed the letter over to my teacher, she was visibly, extremely unimpressed. She no doubt thought our family believed we were above such mundane things like homework. She raised her eyebrow and archly said to me 'Excuses, Roman?'

When I went home that night, Mum asked how it had gone, and I told her the teacher's response. Or rather, I did an impression of her. Mimicking the teachers was my favourite pastime.

Well, that was it. Fuming, Mum got straight in the car, drove back to the school, and had a right go at the teacher!

Some kids might have been extremely embarrassed by this, but I wasn't remotely. I just thought – brilliant! I really understood that Mum was wholly and unconditionally on my side. She had my back. And I was grateful.

There have been so many times over the years when I've had reason to be grateful to Mum.

It was her who first spotted the signs of depression in me.

I was just 15 when Mum realised something was off.

She says that I went from being this full of beans character, who loved entertaining everyone with impressions and jokes, to someone who started opting out and withdrawing from family life. Or I'd get frustrated and short tempered.

I think she was more acutely aware of the signs in me because she'd grown up with her own father, Henry, who'd suffered with depression all his life. I don't think I ever saw Grandad smile, like ever, he was an odd one alright. And an angry, aggressive, violent man. Mum told me about depression and anger issues she was aware of in her family. So she was terrified for me, the idea of that being my destiny, too.

No parent ever wants to think their child needs antidepressants. And Mum now admits that the first time she said those words out loud to my dad, 'I think Ro suffers from depression,' she felt almost guilty suggesting it. She was worried that she would seem like some neurotic parent and landing me with some kind of label I wouldn't want.

Mum knew that it wasn't my life being bad causing the mental health issues, far from it. But she saw my mood swings, and she saw me stepping away from family life and generally acting like a miserable dick. She recognised it wasn't just being a sulky teen. (Though I am sure she'd claim I was that too, of course.)

There was no denying that – despite a great childhood, a great school, great friends – I had these extreme highs and lows that I wasn't always able to deal with. Many times I'd be curled up in bed crying and Mum would be there for me.

She marched me off to the doctor's, but she didn't come in the room with me. She waited outside, she thought it was important I talked to the doctor honestly about how I was feeling. She says she didn't want to put words into my mouth. But sure enough, blood tests confirmed my diagnosis of chemical depression.

I've been on pills ever since then.

Mum cottoned on to the fact that as a kid and teen she would get the most chat from me in the car, while we were sat side by side rather than facing each other. This has actually been proven by psychologists who recommend it as a way of getting kids to open up. I think it works because it made me feel less directly interrogated and more willing to talk. She'd often drive the long way round so we'd have more chatting time. It's so effective I now use this technique myself with my friends, we get in the car or go for a walk. Try it yourself – it works.

It was also Mum who came to my rescue three years ago, when I reached my very lowest ebb. I'll tell you more about that later, but Mum got straight in her car that time and came to save me. I was very lucky my mum called me that day. It could have all gone very differently for me. Life without Mum is frankly unthinkable. She's my everything.

Three random things you might not know about my mum.

- She is very particular about calling people 'artists'. She thinks the term 'singers' doesn't give them enough respect. She's drummed it into me so many times I now say artists too – though admittedly sometimes people think you're a bit pretentious.

- Mum is CONSTANTLY on the go. Whenever we're on the phone, all I can hear in the background is her clattering around, doing chores or walking the dogs while we chat. I often want to shout, 'JUST SIT DOWN WOMAN.'

- To my knowledge, Mum has only kissed one man apart from my dad. She's had two men in her life. Her first boyfriend was Andrew Ridgeley from Wham! And my dad.

THE BIG LIST OF MY LIFE

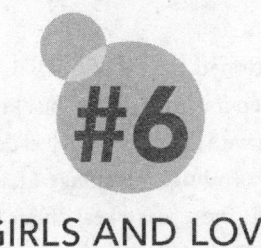

GIRLS AND LOVE

***'The search for the love my mum and
dad have...'***

Even the most mentally well and secure person is going to find the quest for true love tricky at times!

I think Mum always hoped I might be gay and I could avoid some of the heartbreak I've had with women. But whoever you're in a relationship with, there's always going to be a certain amount of conflict, confusion and yes – pain.

Getting together, splitting up, getting over it all and starting again – it can be a proper headfuck for anyone. But relationships are a massive part of being human.

I had my 'sexual awakening', let's call it, watching Kate Winslet as Rose in the film Titanic. I was probably 11, maybe 12. It was the steamy sex scene when Rose and Jack are getting all frisky in the car hiding in the engine room that did it.

Suddenly, playing football with the lads or being glued to endless video games wasn't just what life was all about anymore.

Girls were now officially on my radar.

I've realised that growing up with an extrovert older sister, a very strong-willed mum and my adoring, beloved nan gave me an advantage, because I was used to these big female characters in my life, and I respected them more than anything. There was also Dad's mum Eileen, who I loved. I have all these amazing women's names tattooed on me. So it's not surprising that I wasn't at all shy when it came to girls. Just knowing how to chat to them normally, have a laugh and not feel desperately awkward in their presence was a huge advantage I had over some of the other boys at school. There was a real divide between those who had sisters and those who didn't.

First kiss

My first kiss happened when I was still at prep school. The school was all-boys but there was an all-girls school nearby, and we'd all started checking each other out a bit, but it was all very sweet and innocent back then.

It was that classic thing all kids do at that age, where each boy has to find a girl they're into, and each girl does the same. And you kind of have to pick each other, but it's all communicated in that very mature way – through each other's mates. And there's an unspoken rule that if you're kissing a girl, her friend seems to kiss your mate.

There was definitely a pressure there – who's going to be the first person to kiss? Who's gonna be the first person to do any of that sort of stuff? We'd stand around awkwardly, in our terribly uncool purple blazers, and one of our friends gave his earnest advice: 'You have to go big with your tongue,' he explained to the group, as we nodded knowingly. 'You move it around like it's a washing machine.'

We were all totally terrified of snogging full stop as the week before we'd seen a boy and a girl – both braces wearers – go in for a kiss and manage to actually lock their metallic train track together.

We'd all witnessed how she somehow fell into the boy – I

assume while trying to extract lips – and then one of their mums (I kid you not) had to go in and help separate them. Imagine!

We were scared, but still wanted to get this rite of passage over and done with.

Surprise, surprise, it was me put forward to make the initial approach on some unlucky girl. I was 11 and the poor person and subject of my slobbery, hopelessly amateurish affection went to the local girls' school.

We were all gathered at my mate's house, my friends, her friends, and me – stinking strongly of Ralph Lauren's Polo aftershave, which I must have thought was the height of sophistication back then. I moved in for the lips, with everyone watching.

Having never kissed anyone in my life, it must have been horrendously bad – wet and messy, and I probably had that washing machine advice at the front of my mind. It was horrendous, actually. To that girl now, I'd like to wholeheartedly apologise! But the first kiss was done.

I don't think we ever progressed from there, I was quite immature and naive, and I'm pretty certain we never repeated it again.

But there were other underage fumbles around one friend or another's house. Arguably, I lost my virginity to someone round at a mate's house with everyone watching too and weirdly encouraging it to happen. I say 'arguably' as I genuinely was clueless and not a hundred per cent sure the deed was even correctly committed. It was completely inappropriate.

But it was all very childish. If you 'went out' with someone at that stage, all it meant was that you had their name with a heart next to it in your MSN messenger. (MSN Messenger! Remember that? A true Millennial blast from the past.)

But Mum has always made me believe that women are the superior species, they are much more emotionally intelligent than blokes. And Mum ingrained in me from a young age about respect for women and the importance of consent. I am so grateful she did. I've always looked up to women much more, guys could be such neanderthals.

I remember my Grandad Henry – my mum's dad – handing me a packet of condoms when I was 13. I was so embarrassed I hid them hastily in a cupboard drawer and thought, 'You don't know me at all.'

First heartache

I was 14 when I suffered my first 'break-up'. She was an older girl, well, all of 15, and it was what you'd call a typical 'school romance'.

We were barely even together, it was probably all of four weeks tops, and we only ever kissed each other. But she turned around one day and decided, 'Nah, I don't like Roman after all.'

And for some reason it's the heartbreak that hits me the hardest in my life.

Still, to this day, I see this girl on Instagram and remember the moment she rejected me, and how much it really hurt me realising she didn't want to be with me.

Even now when I listen to the Kings Of Leon album Only By The Night it takes me right back to being 14 and sitting forlornly on the school bus thinking, 'How can I win this girl back?'

The school bus would go past her house every morning, and whenever I listen to that album it brings back exactly those feelings of being hurt.

I can still feel how sad I was, and how I hoped the bus would go past her house and I'd get out and we'd bump into each other. That experience took me a while to bounce back from and I still think about it.

I've met up with that girl once since then. If anyone asks me who *The One That Got Away* was, she's still that person in my head, which might seem weird as it was 15 years ago.

First w*nk

As a teen I must have spent hours on MSN Messenger and on the similarly now-defunct LimeWire, where I normally downloaded porn.

I'd become interested in masturbation and things like that, as teenagers do, and I remember being upstairs giving it a cheeky go for the first time.

Then Mum shouted at me to come downstairs for dinner with my family. I was, ahem, in the middle of 'things' and I'd ignored her for a while.

Until she started yelling ever louder: 'Come on Ro! The food's getting cold! HURRY UP!'

Sheepishly, I went down downstairs, not quite prepared for the full Spanish Inquisition treatment from Mum, who was standing just a metre away from me and peering closely at me. 'Why are you so sweaty, and why are you so red?'

Dad could see I was uncomfortable and, knowing my dad, was quite probably smirking. 'Let him be, Shirlie! Come and sit down, Ro.'

I felt like Dad understood precisely why I was so red and sweaty, and was trying to help me out. Which frankly made it even more cringe for a developing, experimental teen… No kid wants their parents to know about them discovering wanking.

I must have infected so many family laptops over the years with viruses from my dodgy downloaded pornography videos. My parents never bothered blocking any website, or (more likely) actually didn't have the technical know-how. But Mum and Dad finally got me my own laptop though, so they must have got fed up!

At that time I also insisted on having an entirely black bedroom – black walls, bedsheets, black everything which in hindsight probably wasn't the best idea for a teenage boy's room…

One of my most mortifying experiences was Dad actually walking in on me once in the act. Dad always had – and still has – this annoying habit of knocking on the bedroom door… but only right before entering anyway. Like, why bother knocking unless you're asking for permission to come in, and waiting to find out whether now is actually the right time to enter?

So he knocked and failed to wait for my 'nooooo you can't come in!' response and caught me right at it. There I was, sat at my bedroom desk with my knob out in front of the computer screen, halfway through watching some naughty video.

In my complete horror at this rude interruption, I quickly spun around in my swivel office-style chair to try to cover the evidence, but completely unbalanced myself in the process, thus sending the swivel chair and myself – trousers around my ankles, hands still wielding my penis – crashing sideways to the ground. BOOM!

Wanting the floor to open up and swallow me doesn't even cover it.

You'd think most parents at this very sensitive point might choose to discreetly back out the room, apologise, and allow their mortified teenage lad some privacy. You know, some time in which to regain even a morsel of their dignity. But not my father. Oh no. Instead, for the next few seconds, all I heard was Dad's big-bellied laughter as he pointed at me. Pointed at me. Doubling up with the hilarity of it all.

I scrambled to my feet, shouted at him to go away. And asked whether I could have a lock on the bedroom door after that.

As you can imagine, my parents being the bohemian kind they were, they were incredibly open about sex. I don't mean they were busy at it in front of me and Harley – God, no! – but in terms of being able to talk about it there was no awkwardness.

Mum and Dad are like an open house, and I've lost count of the times I've brought back girls who've seen Dad walking around naked. He's one of those people who just doesn't care. And I think the girls quickly learned not to care either. It's hard to shock anyone in our house.

Some people say it's mortifying watching sex scenes and things in front of their parents, but never with mine. In fact, anyone who's watched my dad and I watching TV together on Gogglebox will know what we're like, and how open we are. We all have a laugh about sex and it's certainly not taboo. Which is lovely, actually, knowing I can chat to them about anything has helped me be open in life.

I think the reason Mum always secretly hoped I'd be gay, was not because she was remotely threatened by me having relationships with girls. On the contrary, she's taken me aside before and told me: 'This is as good as you're going to get Ro and you should count yourself lucky.' But I think she would have liked me to have been gay, or just not interested in settling down, so I wouldn't have to go through all the heartbreak of relationships with women. But I dream and hope about raising kids with a woman I love one day. That's the ultimate goal.

First girlfriend

I didn't have a proper girlfriend until I was 16. I was very in love with her and we went out until I was 19.

Now, I know I am very open – and I will happily talk about anything and everything to the nation on radio and TV. But when it comes to girls, and the women I've had relationships with, I am a little more cagey. And I apologise for this, because I promised you this book is about me sharing my life, right?

But it's not fair on the girls to be named, and it's not fair if they're being looked up on the internet because of something in my book. So I'm keeping names and details out of it.

Yet I can tell you that my first real love was a girl I met at college, I was only at this college for a year because I'd got in the band by then (more on that later). But she was my first girlfriend, and I really fell for her. She was the first person I started properly understanding sex with.

They say men fall in love with people like their own mothers. I don't know whether that's true, but my own mum certainly came from a complicated home life with her own parents, so perhaps I have been more drawn towards women who are a little bit vulnerable? Don't get me wrong, when I think about the women I've liked, I've always been attracted to independent women, with strong personalities and lots of confidence, people who have made it on their own.

But often there's a vulnerable background in common.

I've realised, now I'm 29 and have got some life experience under my belt, that I might be attracted to people who I feel I can help somehow.

Most people I've dated haven't been fortunate enough to have had the solid family background I have been blessed with.

THE BIG LIST OF MY LIFE

I know how lucky I am and I've always been keen to bring girls in my life into that and show them that love I've been given. So this girl from college had become part of the family for a while, she was a great person, we had a real connection, and instantly my mum loved her.

She came on holiday with my family and was always at our house. I suppose you could say she had come from a little bit of a broken home, her parents didn't really speak to one another.

But we supported each other in different ways and, in many respects, helped each other to become adults in those formative years. She didn't really know what she wanted to do in life. I helped her to come to the conclusion that she wanted to be a photographer, so I helped her save up and buy her camera.

She was very kind to people, which I liked, and she was very supportive of me when I needed it. But it didn't work out. We fell out of love. We became friends. We grew into adults. We shared so many important experiences but it wasn't to last. Some relationships just don't pan out and you drift in different directions.

I'd say I was a good boyfriend, I'd say I was emotionally available, but I haven't always been perfect. I've made mistakes, like anyone else. There've been times where I've cheated on partners before – and felt horrendous about it. And that ended the relationship. That's life and you go through these things growing up don't you?

Future dreams

I'm currently single. I'm 29. And I long to meet the right person one day.

I'm scared of relationships. But when I'm going out with

someone, I'd say I am full hog into it. I love being with someone in a partnership.

Having parents who met and fell in love so young – Dad was 22, Mum was a bit younger – had made me want that myself.

Dad had seen Mum perform with Wham! on Top Of The Pops singing Young Guns, and always says he couldn't take his eyes off her. She felt equally smitten and said she was going to marry him immediately. Up until then, the only man she'd ever kissed was her first boyfriend, Andrew Ridgeley from Wham! That's mad.

On their very first date to the Camden Palais, Mum was so scared she brought her best mate George Michael – who we called 'Yog', which was his Greek name – along as her wingman, and Dad had to spend the whole night trying to get rid of him! And they've stuck together through thick and thin ever since and remain as loved-up as ever, even nearly 40 years later.

That's quite some record to live up to.

Their strong marriage is something I admire so much. As I've said, as a teenager it was one of my biggest fears, them splitting up. I never wanted Dad to ever do Strictly Come Dancing in case the famous curse struck and it broke them up! And because I've seen how happy and solid they are together, I am always chasing it for myself. It's a huge, huge thing for me, and for Harley too, I think. We're both chasing the relationship our parents have because we can see it's the ideal. Will we ever meet anyone to have that? Who knows.

I've certainly struggled with girlfriends dating, all that stuff. In the past I'll admit I've been an absolute asshole. And I've let work get in the way.

But the one thing I know that I want more than anything in this world is the relationship that I see my mum and dad have.

THE BIG LIST OF MY LIFE

And the thing I most panic about in the future? The thing I most worry about is not being able to have kids when I'm older. I think it's an insecurity that a lot of men actually have, but it's never talked about.

That is honestly my biggest fear in life. And I do talk to my friends about it. I feel my main purpose on this Earth is to make other people, you know? That's how I feel. I'm such a family person.

But I'm also worried that, at this point in time, if I got into a serious relationship, I wouldn't be able to give that person what they deserve in terms of being a proper partner. I'm so focused on work right now, and I'm enjoying that and my life, and don't want to defer from that right now.

I've been on dates with the wrong people sometimes, who've tipped off the paparazzi to be waiting somewhere as we've come outside. I've felt hurt sometimes, but as Dad always says to me, 'And what?' He says you can't take those personally, you have a great life, get on with it and don't complain or say 'poor me'.

I've struggled in relationships in the past, and I still will struggle going forward if I'm totally honest, because I always have this massive fear that there is resentment on my future partner's path.

I mean, I feel I couldn't be with someone that doesn't really work for a living, or have a career and passion themselves, because I'd be so scared that they'd be looking at me thinking, 'Well, it's fine for him because he can get this or he can afford to do this, that and the other.'

So I always try my best to make sure that I'm with someone who I can raise up as much as people on the outside raise me, you know?

I don't want a girlfriend to be in my shadow.

That's a horrible thing that I see with my mum and dad, her sometimes getting ignored and passed over by people when she's out with him.

I don't want it to be like that with my partner. So if anyone comes up to me and praises me for how well they think I'm doing, I'm always keen to point out what any girlfriend is achieving too. I don't want it all to be about me.

I've seen so many asshole people over my whole life, when the celebrities introduce themselves to you, and you're chatting, and they don't even introduce their partner to you.

I've seen that happen up front, many, many times, where people just want to talk to my dad. Mum is fine with that. But I don't want my partner to feel like everyone just wants to talk to Roman. I really don't. I don't want my partner to feel they are any less important than me if they don't earn as much money or aren't receiving as much gratification as I seem to.

I think that's why when I look at girls I've dated in the past, they're people who are busy doing their own thing and they're fucking good at it. That's what I've found really attractive about women in my life so far.

To be totally honest, one of the reasons why I don't really date English girls is because I love it when someone doesn't know what I do for a living or not caring about who I am. I love someone not giving a shit about any of that.

If someone was to speak to my last two ex-girlfriends and ask them why our relationships ended, I imagine they'd say that I was too focused on work, too busy with what I'm doing.

You know, I don't think there's anything fundamentally wrong with being work-focused right now because I am feeling fulfilled and happy.

And that's OK. There's a time for everything.

THE BIG LIST OF MY LIFE

I've learned that a relationship is all about compromise. And it's about finding someone that is your best friend, not about something that you just find attractive.

I'll be totally honest with you, after I lost Joe, I kind of got in this mindset where I felt I'd wasted my time. I am sure many girls feel like that when it comes to guys!

But I felt like I was trying to compromise when I should just be trying to enjoy my life more.

So for now, I'm better off being single.

I could get in a situation where I'm seeing someone but I know I wouldn't be able to give them what they deserve. A girl doesn't deserve to have someone who might be too tired that day to even text them.

But I really hope one day I'll find that happiness with someone. And that the right person comes at the right time for me. Because I am very much a relationship person and I have to have faith that will happen for me. I'm a family person and I can't wait to have my own one day.

FAMILY MATTERS

***'What is nature, and what is nurture?
It's fascinating to go back a generation'***

If my parents shaped the person I've become, then of course their own mums and dads played a vital part in their characters, too. Mum and Dad's upbringing had such an impact on their relationship, with each other and with their kids. Dad wanted to emulate his very loving parents, while Mum on the other hand was certain from a young age that she wanted a very different life and marriage to the one her folks had.

I can see parts of all four of my grandparents' personalities inside me, too. And being aware of both the good – and the bad – has given me some helpful insight. It also makes me question what makes us how we are?

Mum's mum, my nan Maggie – we were so close

I was incredibly close to my mum's mum, Margaret, or Maggie as she was known. My nan. I loved my dad's parents too, but there was something very special about my bond with Nan.

We spent large parts of my childhood living with her, and I absolutely adored her. When Dad was working in LA she came to live with us. It was funny seeing this tough old lady from Bushey being transported to the glitz of LA.

Nan had grown up part of that generation when people didn't know or understand the real risks of smoking, and for as long as I could remember, she had horrendous lung problems as a result.

She would come over to our house about three times a week and I got used to setting up her nebuliser for her, and carefully adjusting it on her face, while we'd sit together watching her favourite TV shows, like The Weakest Link.

She was the first woman outside of our little family – other than Mum and Harley – who I really loved and cared for. She'd had a very tough life, and she was hard as nails. She was sweary and funny and seemed different to other old ladies.

She'd drag me around Costco in Watford with her, haggling over the price of bananas. If we went to stay with her for the weekend, she'd take us to the Harlequin Shopping Centre. She liked to keep it real.

Yog, who was also my Godfather, loved my nan and he'd fly her around the world when my mum went on tour with Wham! To us, Yog was never a world-famous pop star or the best singer-songwriter of his generation or an icon – or any of those other big labels bandied about. To us he was always just 'Yog'.

My parents also flew Nan and Dad's parents all around the world with them when they went on tour in their youth. I think they loved being able to do that for them, showing them all the opportunities there were and letting them share their success.

With Nan, I sat and chatted about everything and anything. We were that close, good mates.

It was always her I spoke to about who I had a crush on, and what I should do about it, and anything else that was on my mind. We had proper conversations about life. If I felt down, I'd tell her.

We've got countless home videos of me pretending to be Frank Sinatra as a kid, doing full performances for Nan. They must have been pretty awful actually, and yet she'd sit there smiling indulgently, lapping them up. That was her era of entertainment. She loved Elvis too, and when she was very sick and didn't have long left to live, she'd tell me not to get sad – because she couldn't wait to go and marry Elvis in heaven.

My grandad, Nan's husband, and my mum's father, was not a nice man at all. He was depressed for much of his life and their marriage had not been a happy one, so I was told. They would shout and swear at each other – and worse. They were like chalk and cheese but couples didn't separate back then. It wasn't really an option.

When Nan was dying, I was 15, and we became her carers until she went into hospital. I remember sitting with her in the ward in her curtained-off little section, trying to adjust the TV screen so she could watch her very favourite show Strictly Come Dancing while she was lying down bedridden. She loved all the dancers and glitz and glamour.

If Nan had been alive I would have definitely tried to get on that show to make her happy.

We were at the hospital a lot back then, we'd visit every day after school.

Towards the very end, I sat holding Nan's hand and she quietly stroked the top of mine with her soft, wrinkled thumb, looked at me and smiled: 'I want to go now, I can't do this anymore.' She was in so much pain.

I said: 'I know, Nanna, I know. It will be soon.'

I could see Grandad had just arrived at the hospital and was sitting outside the room. I asked if she wanted me to bring him in. Her eyes snapped open, 'Why the fuck would you want to do that?' Later, when I told Mum, we had a laugh about that. But at her funeral, it was the first time I'd ever seen Grandad cry. Mum didn't though. She adored Nan and had done so much for her over the years, but Mum is proper tough.

Nan's passing was my first experience of losing someone I really loved. I understood how final it was, death. When someone is gone, they're gone. It was the first time I'd suffered grief. But at that age you bounce back, you carry on going to school and you don't really process it until much later, I think.

But I still miss her.

Mum's dad, my grandad Henry – I didn't feel much

Mum's dad was not a nice man, I grew up not liking him.

Mainly, this was because of what my nan used to tell me – that he would come home with other women, he was violent and aggressive and would literally throw her against the wall or into a door some nights. He was an angry man. And he sounded like a depressed man. Mum grew up fearing him and his moods. I think that's one of the reasons why she was so terrified when she first saw the signs of depression in me.

Grandad wasn't interested in me. I'd go round to their house and he wouldn't even look at me half the time. He'd be sitting in a chair in the corner of the room watching Formula One wearing dungarees with paint splattered all over them. No T-shirt underneath. For some reason, I can still vividly remember he had these really white hairy nipples on display. He was a massive, big geezer, like 6ft 5ins, with these huge builder's hands. And he was a horrible racist. I remember him one time winding his car windscreen down to actually snarl at black people. I was horrified. Poor Mum having to grow up with him.

Towards the end, he'd remember my name and say, 'How's Roman?' but he couldn't even remember Harley's name. He'd just say, 'How's the girl?'

He'd spent some time in prison and grew up in a bad way.

Dad – always the first person to try to understand other people – agreed that Grandad wasn't nice. Yet Dad always tried to have some element of understanding about Grandad's bad behaviour. He would explain to us that yes, Grandad wasn't a kind man, but remind us of all the things he'd been through in his miserable life.

It's sad, but whenever I think about my grandparents now, I always forget about Henry. He ended up living longer than any of the other grandparents, but I just didn't feel much towards him.

Dad's parents, Frank and Eileen – a true romance

One of my biggest regrets in life is that I wasn't there when my dad's parents passed away. I was 18, I had my head elsewhere, and I wasn't in tune with what was going on.

They died in January 2009 within just 48 hours of each other.

My grandad was nicknamed 'Nank' by the family as Harley couldn't say Frank when she was little, and it sort of stuck. He was 79 when he got rushed to hospital with a heart attack. I remember I was out with my friends at the time, and although I cared deeply, and loved him, I was distracted, a self-centred teen.

I always think about that. Why didn't I go to the hospital? Harley did. Why didn't I go with her? Looking back now, that was so stupid and I wish I'd been there.

The reality is that he was out of it by then. We wouldn't have been able to have a conversation. But I wish I'd gone to see him just one last time. Or I wish I'd gone to be with my nan, Dad's mum, and be there for her when she died.

Weirdly, she ended up passing away the next night, just in her sleep. She was 77 and had also been in the same hospital that Nank was taken to, as she was having a heart bypass op herself. When she came round from the op, Dad and Uncle Gary had to break the news to her that Grandad had passed. She was so devoted to her husband that Dad thinks she died of a broken heart.

Everything my dad knows about love was taught to him from his own parents. When I think about true romance, I think of Nan and Grandad.

Unlike my mum's parents, Frank and Eileen had the most loving marriage you can imagine. And I'm sure that's why Dad turned into such a gentle man and caring husband too. And why I want to be the same.

Nan and Grandad had been together since they were teens living in Angel, north London, and Grandad took her to the dance hall for a date. I love driving past it now and thinking of them in their youth.

They were obsessed with each other until the end, they were the only old people I ever saw that would hold hands as they walked together and would still kiss each other. They genuinely seemed to love being together 24/7. How many couples can you say that about? If they ever did sometimes fall out, or bicker, there was still a deep respect for one another there. It never got nasty like with my other grandparents.

Mum said she was always so embarrassed when her parents met Dad's, because her folks were so unhappy in comparison.

Frank and Eileen adored their kids – Dad and Uncle Gary –

and always put them at the heart of the family. It was Grandad who bought Gary his first guitar when he was a kid.

Grandad worked in an industrial printing house and when Dad was 16, Grandad thought he was doing his son the biggest favour ever by getting him a job there too.

For that generation of working-class men, life wasn't about finding self-fulfilment necessarily, you just wanted to earn a living for your family. To look after them.

So Grandad could have been very cross and dismissive when Dad turned around after leaving school and said he didn't want the printing job he'd been offered, he wanted to be a rock star.

Instead of laughing at him for having pipe dreams, Grandad totally supported Dad's hopes and ambitions, and wrote to his printing boss explaining that Dad wouldn't be coming back to work, and that he was going off to become a big pop star. It was totally out of Grandad's world, but he wanted Dad to be happy and put complete faith in him.

They were so open-minded, too. While other people started panicking about AIDS in the '80s, they didn't bat an eyelid about Dad going to the Blitz clubs and having gay mates. Unlike my other grandad, with his racism and bigotry, they were welcoming and respectful of other communities and cultures – and brought up Dad and Uncle Gary to be too.

In fact, they were so chilled out about everything, Dad one time purposely tried to shock his dad. As a sort of act of teenage rebellion once, to get a reaction, Dad went up to his mum's wardrobe, took out her dress, jewellery and even tried to squeeze on her shoes. Then he went downstairs dressed like that and announced to Grandad he was off out.

'Oh,' said Grandad, looking him up and down. 'Have a nice time then,' he shrugged. 'See you later.'

He was just an accepting, lovely man with strong family values and huge amounts of love to give.

He was a proper East End guy. When they later retired to live in Bournemouth, by the seaside, Grandad took a recording of London at night because he missed the sounds of the streets and the city and he couldn't go to sleep without them.

Harley – my big sis has shaped me the most

Unlike me, with my self-doubt and all my ups and downs, Harley is the craziest, happiest person you could hope to meet.

People often ask if I felt pressure growing up, to be successful because of who my parents are. But the real driving force in my life hasn't been living up to Mum and Dad so much, it's been living up to my big sister.

Growing up with Harley, and trying to live up to her, and impress her, became a defining part of who I am.

Harley is now a hugely successful photographer, so you might imagine that she's the quieter one of the pair of us, someone who's happier behind the camera. But that's not the case. Growing up, it was always Harley who was the real entertainer, happiest in the limelight. She was a total extrovert with a naughty streak. She constantly showed off and was a natural little performer.

I was always, always in Harley's slipstream as a kid. Of everyone in my whole life, it's been her who shaped me the most. Even before I reached Reception at school, Harley would make me learn Craig David's songs, or some of Shaggy's raps, and she'd get me to sing all these sexy lyrics, gyrating on the floor banging and slapping my own arse suggestively.

Neither of us had a clue how inappropriate this must have

looked for a five-year-old, but our parents thought it was bloody hilarious. As did Yog. He'd throw his head back laughing with his lovely big smile at all our antics.

Harley, like any typical big sister, could be so mean to me sometimes. I could be a sensitive kid, scared of sleeping alone and easy to wind up.

I remember running into her room in the middle of the night, aged about six, scared from a nightmare, and I'd try to quietly climb into her bed and sleep there to feel safe. She just rolled over, looked me in the eyes and said in a Darth Vader-like voice-hiss, 'What are you doing?'

'Can I just come in with you?' I'd plead, all pathetic-like.

'This isn't Harley!' she'd growl, trying – and completely succeeding – to freak me out.

Still, I'd gladly trot around after her and beg to be in all her big girl games.

She's always had a really strong work ethic, and when she got a Saturday job sweeping hair at a hairdresser's aged 14, it gave me a real worry and fear that she was doing something I wasn't, and I needed to get a job too. Part of me was always a bit jealous because she kind of had this maturity quite early on, she was making her own money and being independent.

Harley has known that I've been vulnerable at times, and needed more support than her and some help with my direction in life, and she's always been there to give that unconditionally. We are both busy and adults making their own way in life, but we will always remain incredibly tight.

Even when we don't see each other for a while, we know that we would drop anything, anytime, to be with each other if needed.

What else could anyone want from their big sister?

THE BIG LIST OF MY LIFE

Uncle Gary – the one I wanted to impress

Uncle Gary needs a special mention because people always want to ask about him because of his Spandau Ballet fame.

He wrote most of the songs for the band and was always uber bright, uber creative and uber talented. He got into a smart and very musical grammar school, Dame Alice Owen's, where he met friends like Steve Norman, John Keeble and Tony Hadley, who he ended up forming the band with before drafting in Dad.

By the time I was growing up, Gary had split from his wife, the actress Sadie Frost, so I didn't see a lot of her at family gatherings. But their son, Fin, my cousin, and I are still close. And when Sadie went on to marry the actor Jude Law, I'd often head over to their house in Primrose Hill to hang out with Fin. Jude would treat us to seeing the first screenings of some of his Hollywood films, like AI and The Talented Mr Ripley, and that was pretty cool as a kid.

Uncle Gary and my dad are very different though. Dad was a homebody, happiest with Mum and us kids rather than being in company. Whereas Uncle Gary's home was often filled with famous people. He's the opposite of Dad, the real extrovert of the family who loves socialising. So if ever we popped into his house he'd be holding court with all sorts of creative characters round the kitchen table – Bill Nighy, Ian McKellen and high-brow theatre types. Gary is intelligent and mingled with them all. Our side of the family were more like the class dunces!

And it was always Uncle Gary's respect and opinions I'd crave the most.

Unlike my parents treating us kids as adults, Gary's attitude and parenting style was more traditional, like 'you're the kids'.

After having Fin with Sadie, Gary went on to marry a costume designer, Lauren. And had three more boys Milo, Kit and Rex. You'd go round to his house and the boys would be playing Mozart on the piano, whereas round at our house you've got Dad telling some crap 'dad jokes' and we're glued to watching the football.

We are quite different as people, and sometimes I haven't felt that connection. I felt a bit inferior, I suppose, that I wasn't worthy of his respect. I wasn't good enough. But he never said that, he was always lovely. It was just that I felt intimidated because he was so smart.

I always had something to prove to Uncle Gary. He was always the one to impress.

All families are like that aren't they, a mixture? You're not always the same breed of character. But at the end of the day we're blood and we love each other very much.

THE BIG LIST OF MY LIFE

WORK

***'There were many setbacks and false starts and
a couple of jobs I really loathed'***

Most of our waking hours are spent working, and it's often so wrapped up in each of our identities. So the impact on work and mental health is huge.

I'm very career-driven and I LOVE my job hosting the Capital Breakfast show every weekday, as well as all the different TV presenting I do.

But it took a lot of hard graft to get there and there were some hiccups along the way…

Being in a band

(The coolest job for any kid and I felt on top of the world…until it stopped and the depression kicked in)

My very first job was being in a band. Yes, that sounds cool I know. And it was! Unlike my sister, Harley, I'd never even had a Saturday job before that.

I was 15 when I got approached by someone from a record management company. They'd seen me and Dad appear together in a TV show called Dangerous Adventures for Boys.

After it aired they got in touch wanting to know whether

I could play any instruments, sing, or if I basically had any musical talent whatsoever?

Well, as it happens, I'd always played guitar and bass guitar. With my parents' backgrounds in pop, there was always an instrument in the house.

Dad taught himself to play guitar, and was the bassist in Spandau. When I was about six he taught me too, he reckoned I had a good ear for it. But then I got into gangsta rap when I was a teen, so lost a bit of interest. But I could certainly play and was keen to pick it up again.

So of course, when I heard there might be the chance to be in a band, I thought, 'Yeah, brilliant!'

When you're entering that world it's like going down a kind of rabbit hole of meeting different people and different music managers and going to auditions, and suddenly, six months after being in the TV show, here I was at just 15 being offered a record deal with Universal.

It was like a 360 sort of deal, where they wanted me to be available to be in any band project that they fancied trying to get off the ground. So if they just wanted a session player for a gig they could ask me, or if they wanted me to write some music, or play in a band, I could do that too. Effectively, I would describe it as being the label's 'bitch'. They'd call – and I'd have to jump.

I was over the moon, naturally. What teenager on Earth isn't going to think 'this is fucking great!'?

Yog asked his lawyers to look over the contract for me and check everything was legit. Here I was signing a record label deal. Suddenly I couldn't give two shits about the fact I was also supposed to be sitting my GCSEs that year.

I remember being totally unfazed going to collect my exam

results. I managed to get an A* in Religious Studies, and I did well in Classical Civilization. For the rest I got straight Cs – apart from that 'U' in maths I told you about. But oh well, who cared? I was gonna be a pop star! I think within two hours of receiving my results I'd probably tossed that results letter in the bin.

Despite going to a prestigious, fancy school, I just felt relieved to be leaving the education system. I was proudly excited that I was already making money and had leapt ahead about five years in terms of where all my peers were career-wise.

Most of my friends were going to do A-levels and then wanted to go to university. It felt like a big decision to be making, and for the first time in my life (but certainly not the last) I went to my parents for career advice.

And they said the same thing that they've always said to me, 'Ro, you've got to do what you love. You've got to do what's gonna make you happy. Are you gonna say no to something and then later regret that?'

My parents always encouraged me: If there's an opportunity there up for grabs – you bloody well take it. I was going to be well paid, and this was what I wanted to do.

In the end, Universal put me with some other lads drafted in from various places, to form a pop band called Paradise Point. It didn't feel like a cheesy manufactured band to me, and we definitely weren't sitting there on stools with mics. All of the other guys were a year older than me, and we were all from just outside London. It was cool.

We didn't have a stylist, we just dressed ourselves in jeans and T-shirts mainly with the odd leather jacket. I still had my hair in a kind of long mop back then, it was a while before I changed that into a quiff.

Dad was friends with Steve Strange, a Welsh singer who was the lead in an '80s band called Visage. Steve also ran a famous nightclub called Blitz in Covent Garden, a legendary place in its day, where Boy George had been the cloakroom kid and even David Bowie would perform.

Blitz had long shut down by the time we came on the scene, but Steve was running club nights, often with drag queens, or really 'out there' artists, and he set us up with different venues in London.

My parents came to our first gig, but I didn't invite any of my school mates at that point. The audience was packed, yet I don't remember feeling nervous at all. The music started up, the synth kicked in, the strobe lights began, and my heart was pounding with excitement and adrenaline – it was fucking awesome.

I felt completely certain in that moment – THIS was what I wanted to do with my life. We played more gay bars in those two years than I've ever been to since. The crowds were always so honest, had so much fun, were so open to creativity. They were unbelievably welcoming to this bunch of young kids.

I loved playing to an audience where the vibe was so positive, there were never any fights or that testosterone antsy vibe you can get in straight clubs. I'd be playing and watching a 7ft drag queen dancing to our pop music, and it was amazing.

I'll blow my own trumpet here, but we were a really good band to see live. Honest we were. And while we never released a single, we were building a decent fan base as a 'teen live pop band'. We were credible, I thought.

The label was offering to pay to have us make a video for one of our songs, Run In Circles, but I was quite savvy with making videos and offered to do it myself. Why spend money on it? I knew I had the skills.

THE BIG LIST OF MY LIFE

So, in my parents' living room – they helped out with a few props I think – I got the cameras set up and directed and edited the whole video. It turned out great. And Mum, bless her, made us all sandwiches.

We put our hearts and soul into that band, and normally went out flyering ourselves, we were living in each other's pockets and I loved those boys.

For two years we wrote songs, supported different artists – like Ellie Goulding, Olly Murs, Jessie J, and Peter Andre one time at Rochester Castle – that was a fun gig.

We were driven around in limos sometimes, but normally we were setting it all up ourselves, piling into my mate Jordan's little Mini Cooper with the various equipment.

But we also had times when we played and literally NO ONE turned up. We'd say to the venue, 'just wait 10 minutes please, just wait another 10 minutes', and if still no one showed, we'd just shrug it off and tell ourselves it was a 'rehearsal'.

But they were all flying hours, that's what we called them. The chance to get out there and practise and notch up that performing experience under our belts. I never saw it as having a bad day. It's just something that you learn from. I was having the time of my life. It felt grown up, we were getting paid monthly, and we were living the dream.

I never ever wanted the band to stop. But it all came to a shuddering halt when I was 18. I suppose I should have seen it coming.

With a new band you can either release some material, some singles, then an album, or you can wait and build up all these flying hours to create as much hype as possible and then release something.

So we'd got to a point where we'd been playing with each

other for three years, we'd built a fan base, we'd built relationships with important players in the business, and we'd written an album worth of songs.

We just weren't sure how to progress to the next stage.

The Universal contract was coming to an end, but we had talks lined up with Sony, who were keen to poach us.

But Cameron, the lead singer, just turned around one day and said, 'I don't want to do it anymore.'

Cameron's background wasn't the same as mine, his folks were more conservative. And fair enough, his dad wanted him to go to university and become an accountant, or something respectable with a solid and reliable career ahead.

Cameron rang us all individually on the phone to break the news.

'But it's all going so well,' I pleaded with him, not believing he actually wanted it to end. How could he? We were having the time of our lives.

As Cameron was breaking this bad news to the rest of us, we were literally standing on Kensington High Street about to go into a meeting with Sony. We were expecting to do a new deal with them.

'What the fuck are we gonna do?' I thought helplessly. We couldn't go into a meeting missing the lead singer. It felt like we had nothing. You can't just swap in a new singer. We were a team.

I felt like we were on the cusp of something, and the band had been my whole future. But without a lead singer we couldn't carry on. We didn't consider just getting a new one, it doesn't work like that. Frustration and feeling absolutely gutted doesn't even begin to cover how I felt.

That was the first time in my life where everything just came crashing down around me. It was the first time in my life where I'd experienced a total change in the script. 'Hang on a minute,' I remember thinking, 'this isn't how it's meant to go?'

That day all the boys just walked off our own ways, deflated and dejected, and none of us really had the maturity to handle it or know what to do with ourselves.

I came home, where I was still living with my parents, and I remember just sitting on the end of my bed and experiencing for the first time what I'd describe as a proper depressive episode.

####

'I had piled all my eggs in one basket – and it was gone. For the first time in my life I couldn't just wing it, and I had genuinely no idea what to do next'

####

Although I'd been taking tablets for depression for three years by now, and knew I had the condition, I hadn't until this point ever felt such an almighty downer like this.

Sitting on the end of my bed I just cried and cried nonstop. Mum and Dad would come in to check on me and all I could do was sob, 'What am I going to do?' I had no idea about what might come next for me. I had no band. No job. I hadn't managed to last in education. There were no A-levels to fall back on, there would be no university for me.

I had piled all my eggs in one basket – and it was gone. For the first time in my life I couldn't just wing it, and I had genuinely no idea what to do next.

I could tell Mum and Dad were seriously worried.

I felt so low that I stopped eating. I got really skinny. I wouldn't describe it as having an eating disorder, I wasn't purposely starving myself. I just had no appetite for food or life and certainly no appetite for laughter.

And I went into a shell of not wanting to do anything, not wanting to see anyone and not wanting to go anywhere.

My first taste of 'normal' work

(I'd drive to work in my little Vauxhall Corsa, shut myself in a cupboard for a nap on my lunch break, do a shift and come home)

When I was feeling depressed, I couldn't face socialising. But I did start going to the gym a lot – lifting some weights, getting rid of some pent-up frustration, just for something to do with myself.

I decided I didn't want to do anything to do with the media or being in the public eye. I was embarrassed about failing in the band. So eventually, after moping around for a few weeks at home, I thought I'd get a job in the gym.

It wasn't uplifting and certainly not rewarding, but I needed to earn some cash somehow and give myself a reason for getting up in the morning.

So I took on some shifts at the local gym. Mainly, I was spending the days just cleaning the equipment. Wiping down rowing machines and cleaning other people's sweat off the weights and treadmills. I was also tasked with cleaning the toilets.

Dad, bless him, would sometimes pop by to say hello. Even then he couldn't help trying to encourage me. 'Ro, that is the shiniest, cleanest treadmill I've ever seen!' I could see he was trying to make me feel better, but it didn't really lift my mood.

I seemed to spend hours giving elderly people instructions on how to use the equipment, doing endless inductions for new starters.

I took some qualifications in Personal Training, but it felt totally surreal to have left this amazing lifestyle of being in a band to doing a normal, everyday shift job and being paid the minimum wage. Welcome to the real world, I told myself glumly. What a spoiled dick. For nine months I worked at the gym. And my mental health was not good.

I was desperately embarrassed by my former failings. I thought I'd somehow let down my family name, and people would assume I'd had every advantage and yet still managed to fuck it all up. It was a reality check alright and I was struggling to get my bearings.

This is what life is, this is what normal people do. I was trying to buck myself up, I knew I was lucky, privileged, had nothing at all to moan about, but it's hard to reason with depression, it's hard to be logical when your brain is in a funk.

I missed the band horribly. Those boys had become my life and close mates, but we all drifted. We had a few meet-ups here and there, but the friendships faded away once we'd no longer got any shared purpose. I think seeing each other made us remember the failure and the boys went and found work outside the entertainment and music industry, and we all kind of lost touch.

I never picked up my guitar again after that, it just made me feel sad and reminded me of my failings.

My parents were worried about me. They wanted me to just be happy, after all. Like most mums and dads do. And I had a girlfriend at the time who was kind and supportive. I felt like a fraud. I was stuck in a gloom. My life wasn't going how it was supposed to go. In later years I now know this precise feeling – like your life is simply not going how you want it to go – is one of the unfortunate reasons why so many young men take their own lives.

I knew I had to pick myself up and start all over again.

And then a new opportunity came my way…

Modelling

(I was doing well and landing work but at the same time, it was killing my soul)

It was when I got really, really skinny that I was scouted for modelling.

By the time I was 18 I'd reached 6ft, and by the time I was 20 I was 6ft 2in, so I'm quite tall but I wouldn't say I was ever naturally thin.

As a teen I'd always had a bit of puppy fat, but it hadn't really bothered me, if I'm honest. I was always confident enough about how I looked without beating myself up.

But I started working out excessively after the failures of the band, because it made me get an endorphin rush afterwards. Then, when you start seeing changes in your body, you see abs developing and your arms get bigger, you get a little bit obsessed with it all, and I knew that I was doing it all because it was a coping mechanism after what happened with the band.

It was my way of dealing with that crushing disappointment.

It was when I was walking down Oxford Street in central London during this time of feeling like I'd lost my way that someone came up to me with a flyer asking if I'd thought of modelling.

It was a scout from one of the smaller agencies, I can't remember which one. But with my height and gaunt looks they must have seen some potential.

I put the flyer I'd been handed in my pocket and went home that night and told Harley what had happened. By this time my sister was already carving her own way in her career as a successful fashion photographer, and doing really well.

'You really want to sign with these people?' Harley quizzed me that evening, inspecting the leaflet. She too had been worried that I'd seemed so despondent recently.

'Well, I haven't signed anything and they haven't actually asked me to do anything,' I shrugged.

'Right, well you're not going with them, I'm going to set you up and sort this out,' said Harley.

It was the first time Harley had stepped in and been like a mother figure to me, or like the first time we'd connected as adults together, instead of kid siblings taking the piss all the time. Mum and Dad were in America for a few months and Harley took it upon herself to look after me in their absence.

She knew how upset I was about the band, and she wanted to help me. So the very next day Harley marched me back into Covent Garden and into the reception of Models 1. As a photographer herself, she knew her stuff, and Models 1 is a massively successful agency in Europe. All the big fashion houses and magazines use the people on their books, and some of the original supermodels like Yasmin Le Bon and Linda Evangelista were represented by them too.

Harley shoved me into the reception area and was straight to the point: 'His name's Roman – and he's available for work.'

She introduced me to people who were all very nice and lovely and I was grateful she'd taken over and was pushing me in a direction.

They took my measurements – I had a tiny 26-inch waist at this point – made me take my top off and took some Polaroids. Sure, I felt a little bit self-conscious, but because I was depressed I didn't feel I had much to lose. Why not go for this? It seemed fine.

They took me on their books, and I found myself signed to the biggest modelling agency in Europe. We went home and celebrated a bit that night with a few drinks and some pizza.

####

> **'Being so restrictive with my diet and working out wasn't so great for my mental health. Neither was being in constant scrutiny for how I looked'**

####

I'd never wanted to be a model, but I was cheered up when I found out how much money I could earn – it was thousands of pounds if I could land a big campaign – definitely much more than I was being paid for a shift at the gym.

Within two weeks of that initial meeting I was signed up to be the face of Topman, the male counterpart of Topshop, which at that time was a huge high street name with a flagship store on Oxford Street. Within a few more weeks, there was my mug on massive posters plastered all over central London!

I was still in a depressed state, I'd say, and missing the band.

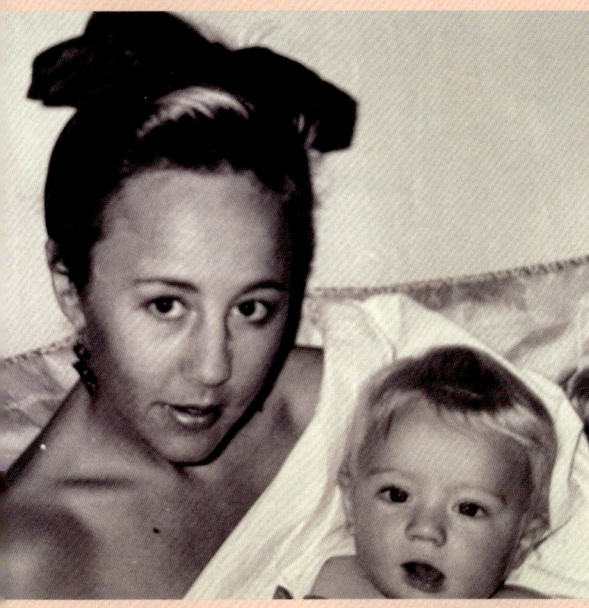

Mum says that I was born Superman-style with my arm raised above my head! Mum and Dad's parenting style was definitely 'bohemian' – but they are the best thing to happen to me

With Dad *(right)* on what looks like my first birthday. Dad is very OCD when it comes to birthday celebrations – he stands there with a big bin-liner to collect the wrapping paper

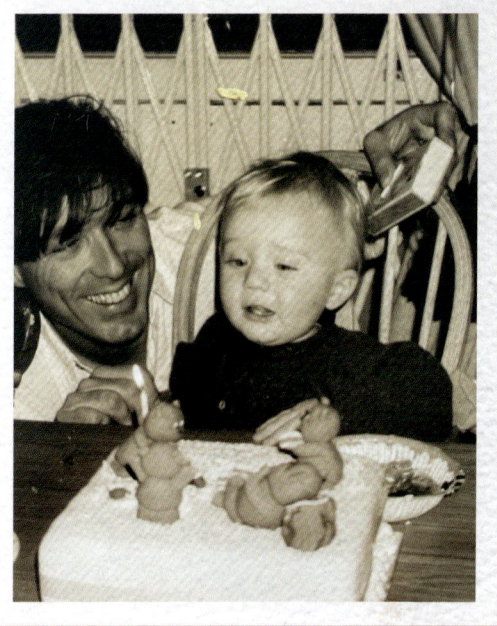

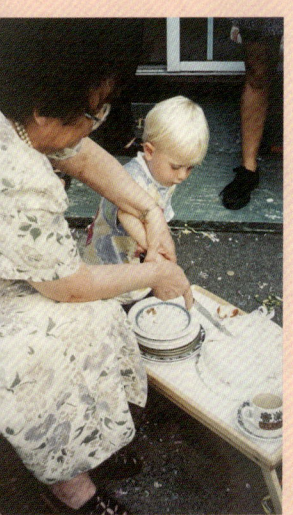

Early days with Nan Maggie. We were always so close, we would sit and chat about everything. When I grew up, we had proper conversations about life

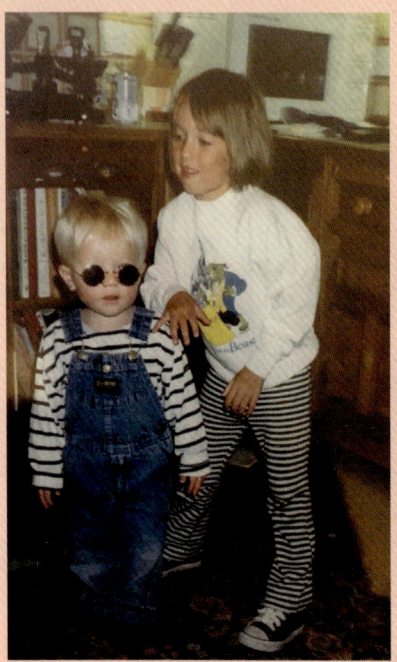

The future's so bright... joking around with big sis Harley. When I first arrived on the scene, it didn't seem like she was keen on sharing the limelight or our parents' affections with little old me – but she got over that!

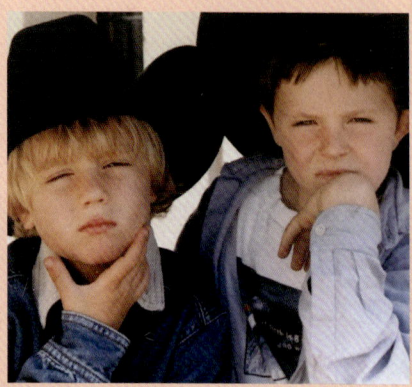

Howdy partner. Dressing up as cowboys with my cousin Fin. Friends loved coming to our house because Mum and Dad were so laid back and didn't have a big set of rules

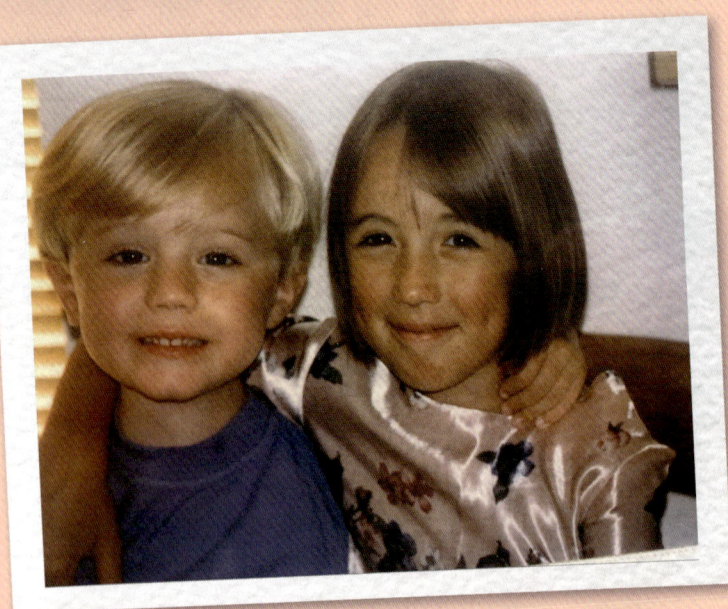

All smiles with Harley. I was always, always in Harley's slipstream as a kid. Of everyone in my whole life, it's been her who shaped me the most

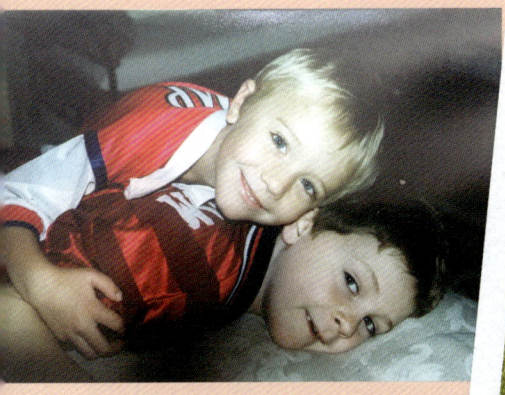
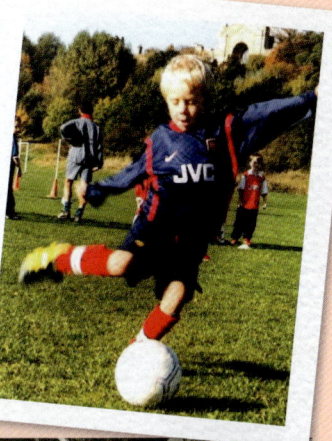

Messing around with a mate and *(right)* about to score a great goal (I hope!) I loved wearing the colours of my beloved Arsenal

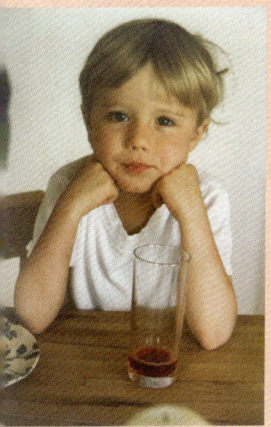

Six years old and not looking best pleased with life. Maybe someone had been drinking my Ribena...

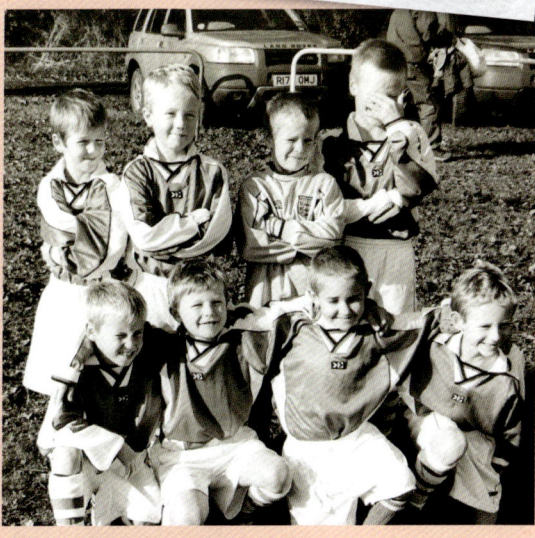

Team shot. At weekends and in the summertime I played football at Alexandra Palace, or Ally Pally as it's known – my first taste of the game I'd grow to love

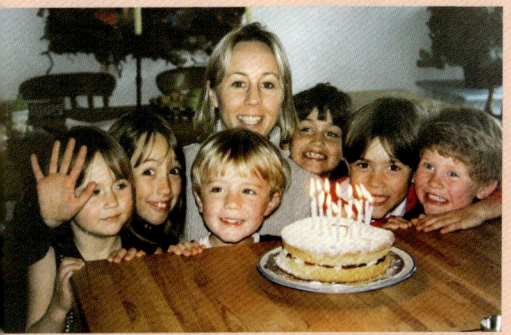

I never went without anything I needed, there were always Christmas and birthday presents and Mum always joined in the fun when she could

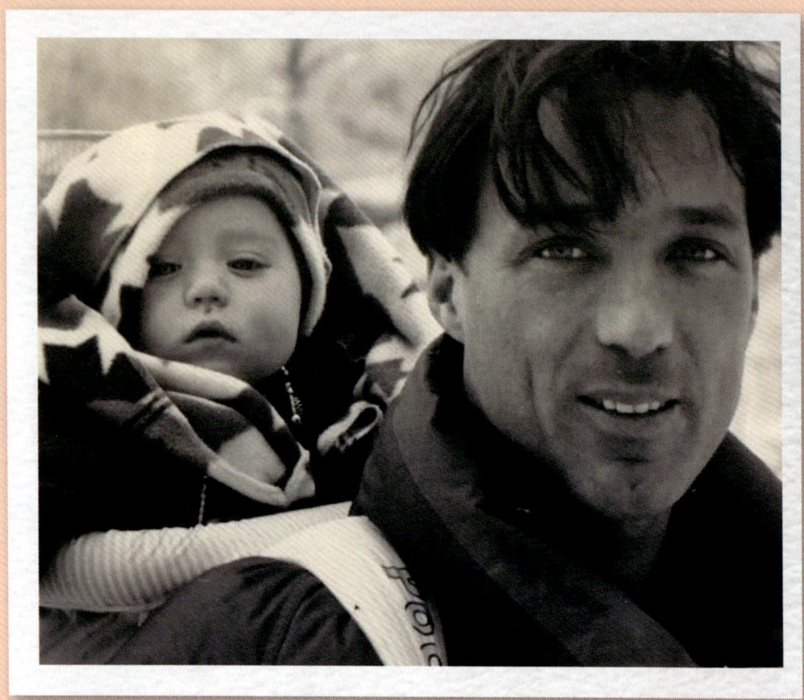

Dad is my hero and my best mate and we have always been insanely close. I am absolutely blessed that we have one of the best father-and-son relationships of anyone I know

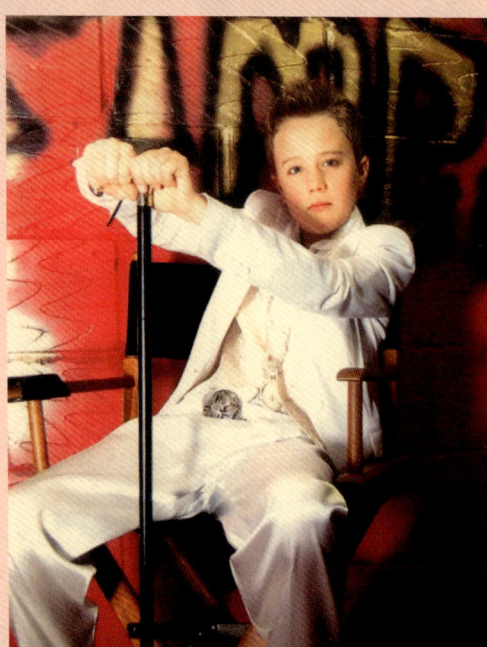

I was such a little entertainer when I was young, I'd be in the middle of the floor in my element holding court, and loving every minute of it

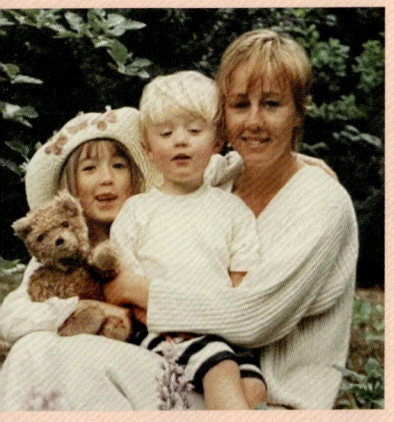
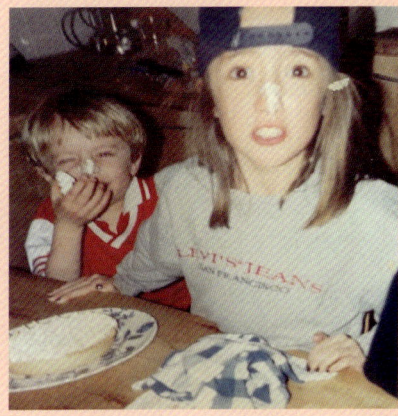
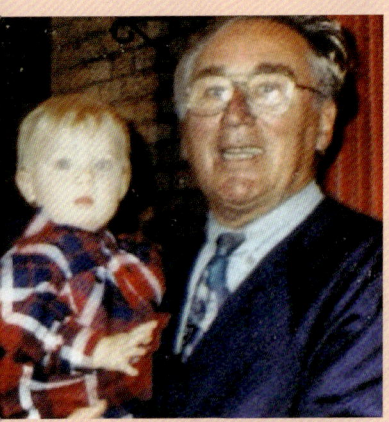
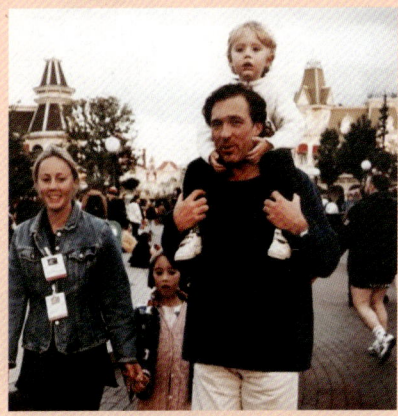
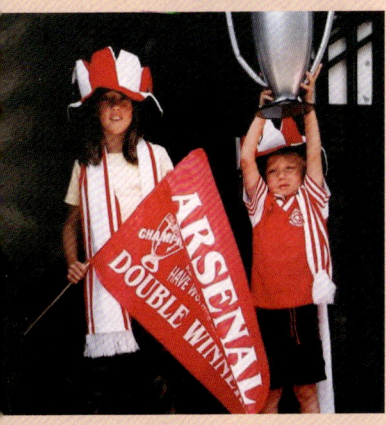
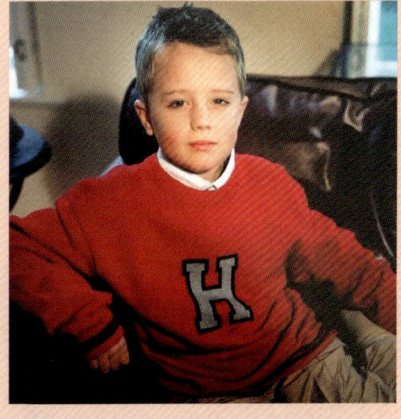

had such a happy, carefree childhood. *(Clockwise from top left)* with Mum, Harley and our teddy bear; messy kitchen time with my sis; on Dad's shoulders on a day out; looking all serious and smartly-dressed; celebrating Arsenal's 'Double' and with Grandad Frank or 'Nank'

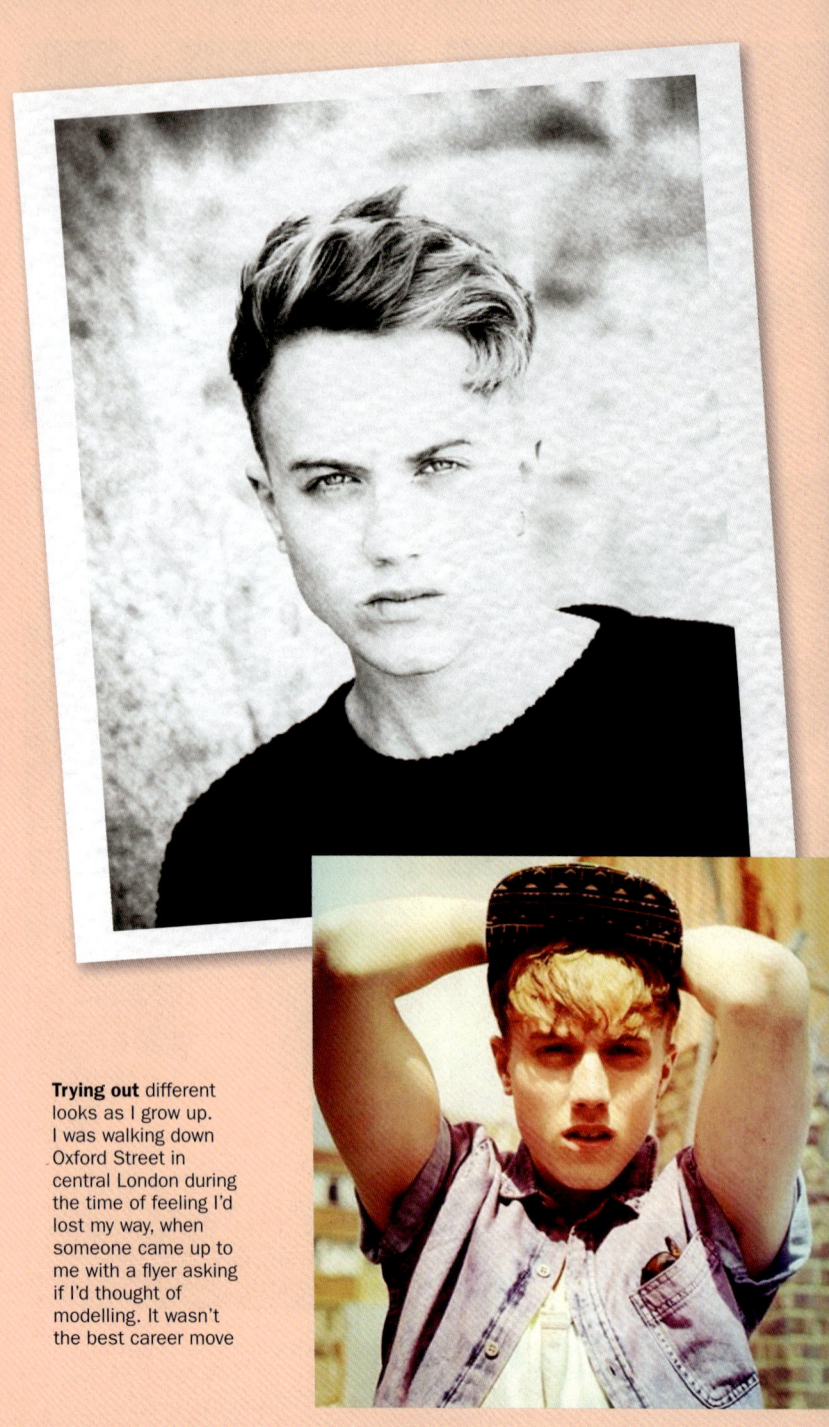

Trying out different looks as I grow up. I was walking down Oxford Street in central London during the time of feeling I'd lost my way, when someone came up to me with a flyer asking if I'd thought of modelling. It wasn't the best career move

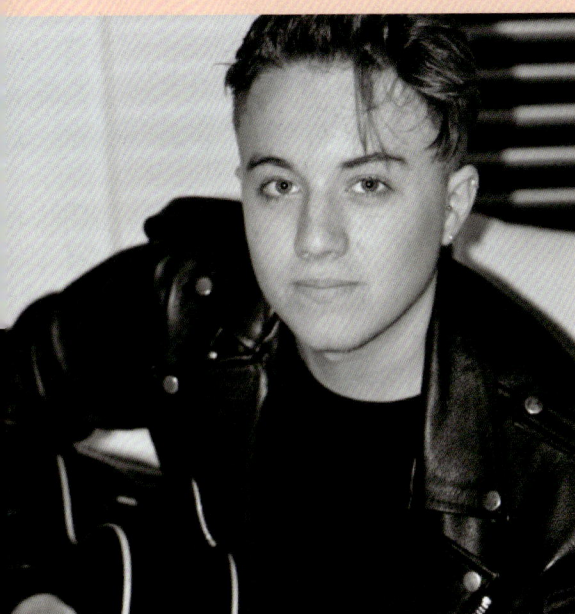

Paradise lost. I loved being in a band and never wanted it to stop. But it all came to a shuddering halt when I was 18

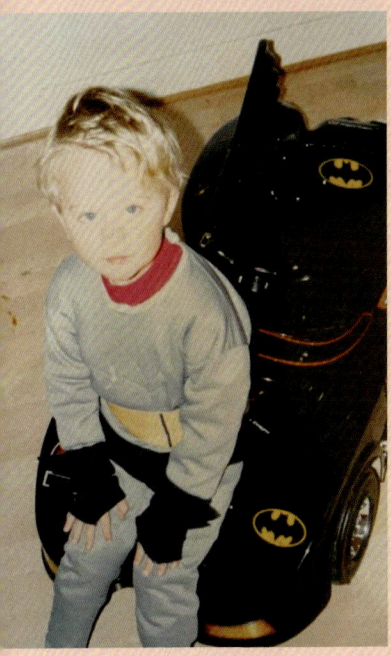

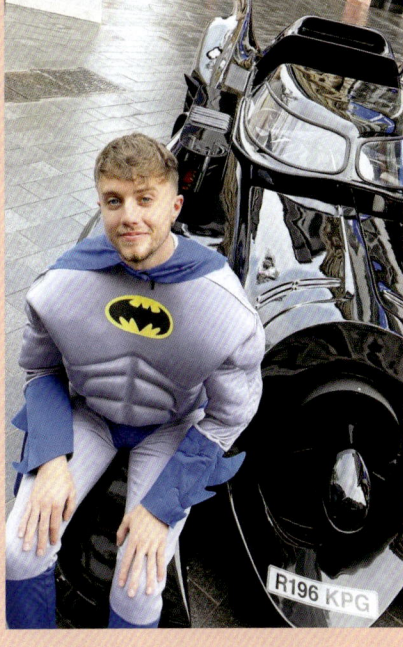

I was so obsessed with Batman as a kid. I had the wallpaper, the duvet, the toothbrush, everything. And thanks to Yog, I had my own bat cave too. I was more than happy to get my Batman kit on again – it brought back some happy memories

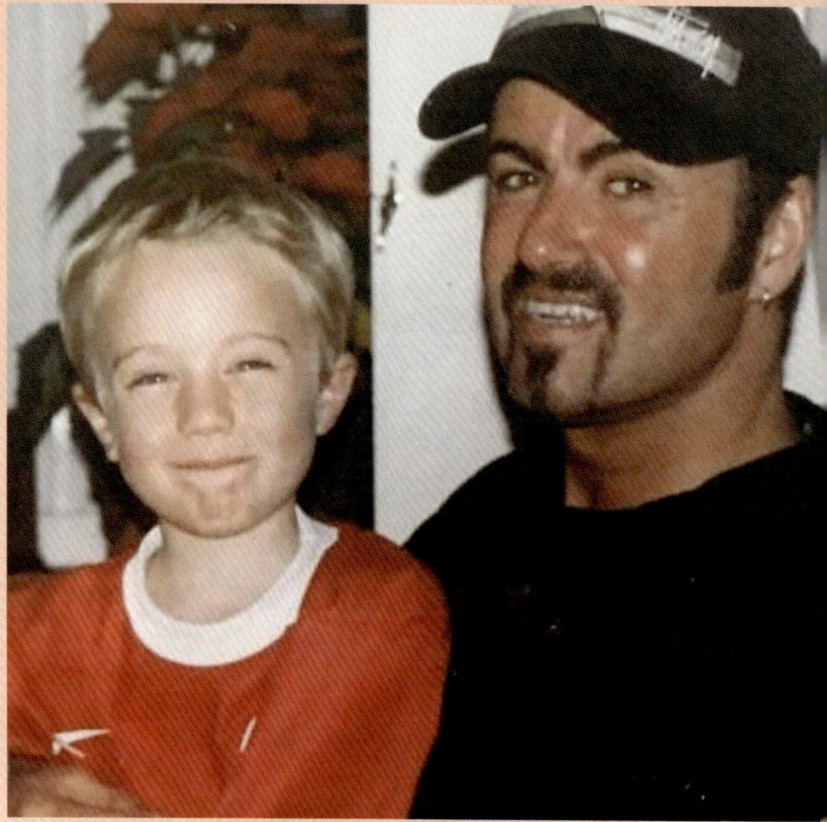

I had such happy times with my Godfather Yog. When I told him Michael Owen was my favourite player, he bought me a Liverpool shirt, which I'm wearing here

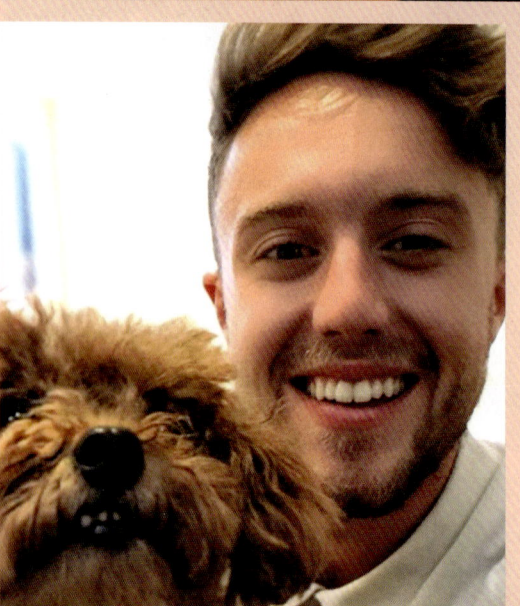

We had dogs in our house throughout my childhood. Here I am with Iris – a miniature poodle my mum and dad saved. Iris is a regular on Celebrity Gogglebox!

I was on my medication – I'll always be on my medication – and I felt a bit of a fraud calling myself 'a model'.

It required absolutely no talent or creativity, but it masked a bit of that feeling of failing that I had.

But as I started working – going to castings, meeting directors, walking catwalks, posing at shoots – I was quickly drawn into what I call the 'wormhole' of modelling.

In my opinion, it's the most fucked-up industry in the world.

I thought the music industry was bad, my experiences with the band and the labels had left me with a bitter taste. But it turns out I just went into another place that was even worse and more depression-inducing than anywhere I'd worked before.

When you're a model, everyone knows you're effectively a human clothes rail. But you're not necessarily treated as a human being.

I was doing well and landing work but at the same time it was killing my soul. I had to work out constantly – often twice a day – to look a certain way and keep that 26-inch waist. I probably weighed around 65 kg, nothing for my height.

So I'd wake up and make porridge in the mornings and that would be my only carbohydrate quota for the day. I'd have a protein shake for lunch and then some bland grilled chicken and vegetables for dinner. Any beers with the football boys had to go out the window as I couldn't afford the calories or risk any bloating on my belly.

Being so restrictive with my diet and working out wasn't so great for my mental health. Neither was being in constant scrutiny for how I looked. I think men don't often talk about their problems with body image, and we don't acknowledge the hang-ups we have, and that in itself becomes part of the problem.

Men can feel just as insecure as women can, especially in this day and age when you feel you're supposed to look as buff as anyone on Love Island or social media.

It wasn't healthy mentally or emotionally, but I became locked in a cycle of denying myself things. It was like I'd worked out the formula they needed and kept getting work. I worked for ASOS, Tommy Hilfiger and Versace.

I was travelling all over the world, getting big catwalk shows, and it was like I was being rewarded by having this existence of denial.

I was asked to go out to Italy and live there for six months. Weirdly, I was invited out for dinner by Donatella Versace, who wanted my sister and me to join her and Lady Gaga. Donatella cancelled at the last minute, but can you imagine how random that evening would have been?!

You'd get stuck in a room with Italian women scrutinising you. You had to walk around with your 'card' which basically becomes your whole identity. My card had my picture of my face on it, my name and my measurements.

You'd walk in, the casting people don't even say hello to you half the time, and you'd hand over the card to a panel of maybe six people. They're all sitting there, watching you, it's like being up in front of the judges of X Factor or something.

They look at the card, maybe ask you to walk about a bit. 'Can you take your top off?' 'Can you strip down to your pants?' You walk about some more, then they say you can leave.

Sometimes it would be more like the TV show The Voice, where the judges have to 'pick you'. So you'd stand there waiting to see if anyone would put their hand up for you. And even then it wouldn't necessarily be picking you to hire you for the job, it would just be to come back for a second casting another day –

or to peer closer at your card. Other times you'd be dismissed and then you'd just have to wait to see if you get the crucial call back.

You learn all sorts of negative things about your looks that in any normal job would never cross your mind to think about. I got lots of pointing at my nose, which apparently is 'Mediterranean'. I learned that my hips – which I'd always just appreciated were strong and sturdy for playing football – are actually 'very wide for a man'. I was told my legs were oddly long and my body weirdly short. Erm, thank you for that!

It's literally like being treated as a piece of meat. Or some alien from outer space who's been stuck in a zoo, while people dissected me. Day in, day out. You're treated like cattle. Like you're something that's come in the room stuck to the bottom of their shoe.

My look was fairly androgynous, feminine even. On the gay scene I'd be described as a 'twink'. Twinks are young looking, skinny and generally hair-free. I honestly had almost no facial hair until I was in my late 20s and I went into the jungle for I'm A Celebrity.

When I look back at the pictures modelling, doing the funny raised eyebrow expression they always wanted me to do, I can't see myself at all. I don't recognize any part of me.

People say, 'Oh modelling is creative, you create looks and moods.' But that wasn't my experience at all. It was just 'do this look' and get on with it. Pose, eyebrows, pose, eyebrows. If you were having an iffy mental health day anyway, let me tell you, times like that could become a massive bloody dent in your self-esteem.

I became self-conscious about smiling and laughing because that wasn't what they wanted. For years I convinced myself I must have really bad teeth. It was all 'be brooding, be intense'. Which really isn't me. I love smiling and joking. But looking back, no wonder I wasn't enjoying myself spending all day long 'brooding' away like that.

Then, in the evenings, you'd have to go to parties. Fancy places like the Saatchi Gallery, the Truman's Brewery or some swanky London hotel opening. I didn't want to be there. I'd frequently get both gay men as well as predatory older women trying to chat me up. I'd normally drink a Diet Coke and get the hell out as quickly as I could.

I knew it was part of the job to flirt, that was how to get hired, whether it was with directors, photographers or people from the agencies. The boys that flirted were the ones who went to parties, and the ones who went to parties were the ones who got the jobs. I didn't want to do the flirting, but I know how to chat to people and make them laugh, that I could do. But I'd feel horribly uncomfortable if someone passed something and held my hand for too long, or pressed their leg against mine. I know what was going on and I wasn't up for it. I was constantly having to tell guys 'I'm straight' because they just wouldn't believe it from the way I looked.

My parents were so open-minded about heterosexuality and homosexuality growing up it wouldn't have mattered to them at all if I was gay. I'm very comfortable in knowing what I like, but it's not men. Not like that anyway.

It's well established in that scene that if you slept with the 'right people' you'd get more work. I was never going to go down that route, though I know people who did. I know straight guys who sucked dicks thinking it would lead to work. And I don't judge them. It was fairly standard practice and quietly accepted as just what happened.

THE BIG LIST OF MY LIFE

The whole experience of modelling was weird and degrading. I knew it wasn't normal for an 18-year-old guy, and I knew it wasn't what I wanted to be doing. In the band we'd been a team, working collaboratively. So being on my own, and being someone's bitch for hire, was awful. But for two years that was my life.

Did I have any pleasure seeing my campaigns? Seeing my face on adverts? Nah. Not really. I was relieved to be working but I wasn't proud of anything I was achieving. People might point at a picture and say, 'Look Ro, there you are!' but I'd just keep up my mask of someone who was doing OK, when in reality I was just numb inside.

Looking around at the other models I worked with, I think everyone felt a bit dead inside. People weren't eating properly or taking care of themselves. Being surrounded by other people who were numb to the world wasn't good for my mental health.

I also knew modelling had a shelf life, and I didn't know where the fuck I was going.

My parents were living in LA for a bit at this point, so if I wasn't travelling around on jobs I'd often be at home alone, watching endless films and crying because I was desperate to be making creative things too.

I didn't tell my family or friends how miserable I was. I was too proud. They all thought I was OK. I was making money, after all, and I had work. I didn't want to admit how worthless I felt and that I was hating every minute.

The straw that broke the camel's back for me was one time when we were rehearsing for a catwalk show back in London and an Eastern European girl fainted on the runway during the practice. She was painfully thin and had prominent veins, clearly she was not a well girl and not fit to be working.

As soon as she swooned to the ground I rushed over to see if she was OK. I tried to get her to eat something but she refused. I ended up slipping some sugar into her water bottle and coaxed her to take some sips.

Then this angry Italian guy, the show director, rushed over. 'What's going on?' he barked at us both. 'She needs some help!' I argued, gesturing at this poor, underweight girl heaped in a right sorry state on the floor.

Instead of showing her some sympathy or offering her any help, he just lost his rag. 'What's going on?' he screamed at her. 'You're so selfish. You're making this all about you,' he carried on. It was at that point – hearing him berate her for being 'selfish' as she drifted in and out of consciousness – when I just flipped.

I shouted at him. 'You are encouraging this behaviour! Like this isn't right. She shouldn't have been hired in the first place.'

I firmly believe that by hiring people like this, you're telling them that they're right for the job and you're creating a terrible pattern.

The angry Italian man looked straight at me and then slapped me across the face. I was fuming, but I didn't retaliate. Dad had drummed it into me throughout my youth that I was never to get into fights. And I knew this man wasn't worth it. And neither was shitty modelling. I was 21 and I collected my bag and coat and I just walked out that room.

I rang my agent as soon as I was outside and told her that was it. I can't even remember whether they tried to persuade me to carry on because I'd told them my decision and then put the phone down and walked away.

I'd made up my mind and my modelling days could very much fuck off.

I was DONE.

THE BIG LIST OF MY LIFE

My lucky break – finding my feet

(I didn't know it at the time but the young guy I'd helped out in the bar, Johnny, was the son of a broadcasting bigwig at Capital called Richard Park)

Quitting the job I loathed was liberating. But what next?

I found myself going back to work in the gym. It was the only alternative career I knew. I felt so lame in the uniform – shellsuit black bottoms and a T-shirt with a collar. I wasn't fulfilling any expectations I had of myself.

Meanwhile, I was watching Harley's career going from strength to strength. She was a successful celebrity portrait photographer, she had her own car and a house in London. And here I was back at Mum and Dad's on a shift rate. All my friends from school who had gone to uni now seemed way ahead of me.

A particular low point was going to pay for my lunchtime sandwiches at Sainsbury's and having my bank card rejected. I was only trying to buy a meal deal. It was humiliating.

I had absolutely no life plan, and found myself in the same position I'd been in two years earlier when the band had failed. Crying on my bed. With Mum worried and trying to talk to me.

'What is it you'd really love to do, Ro?' she gently asked. 'Forget about the money. What are the things that make you happy in life? Try and find some work doing that.'

Mum was right. I needed to think about all the things I enjoyed doing and try to earn a living that way. I'd been handed the band on a plate, I'd been handed the chance to model on a plate. But I knew that I had to do the next thing on my own. Get over myself. Stop thinking everything was fucked and over and make something actually happen.

With Mum's advice ringing in my ears, I thought hard about it, and I realised the things I loved doing were making videos, being creative in some way, and talking about football. I was obsessed with Soccer AM, the Sky Sports show. It's fast and funny and full of banter, and all about football – what I would have given to be presenting that!

I set my sights on landing a job at Sky Sports, and I emailed them, plus every single sports outlet I could think of, sending them a very basic CV and a begging letter. I just wanted to be part of something and have a purpose, and a foot in the door, I didn't care if I was making the tea.

I asked Dad if he knew anyone – I was long past being proud and would happily have let him give me a leg-up if he'd known the right people.

But he didn't.

His world was too different.

So I kept working in the gym during the day, and I bought a camera to film at home. I'm quite savvy with YouTube and KSI – one of the biggest YouTubers on the planet – went to my school.

I took all sorts of random jobs making little films for companies, I was head of video content for the handbag designer Lulu Guinness at one point. And I said to Harley if ever she needed help on a shoot, or to be a videographer, or to edit anything at home, then I would do it. I taught myself all the skills to create bits of content in my bedroom, and picked up little freelance jobs for anyone who needed help making an online video.

'You've got to push yourself, show them what you can do,' encouraged Mum.

I love YouTube and the fact it gives anyone a chance to

express themselves however they want to. You can make people laugh, you can question things, you can learn. As a creative platform, how sick is that?

So with a job at Soccer AM clearly not forthcoming, I thought, sod it – I'll just make a football show on YouTube. I called it Pitch Invasion TV (because calling things 'TV' even when it was online and not actually on TV was all the rage at the time). You can still watch it now if you want to Google it and have a giggle…

####

'A comedy rap I made with my mate Jordan, FIFA 14, went viral, and then suddenly people were noticing me more and asking for me to make content'

####

In the beginning I'd record reviews of matches, I'd talk about players' tactics, make up comedy raps and get all my mates involved. I even had Mum on there wearing a Lionel Messi mask.

It was just from my bedroom or Dad's office but one time I created a whole set using a load of football shirts and flags. I even got in touch with an animator to make an intro for me. I threw the kitchen sink at it, basically, trying to make it work.

I reached out to celebrities and ex-footballers, saying I'd come and interview them, because I knew the benefit of doing cross collaborations, and if they were posting the interviews and stuff online too it would mean more hits and coverage coming our way. I just wanted to create something fun and a bit different. I started promoting it through Twitter and Instagram.

A comedy rap I made with my mate Jordan, FIFA 14, went viral, and then suddenly people were noticing me more and started coming and asking me to make content for them.

One guy wanted me to make a video for a silly slot called 'football pick-up lines', which basically involved me wearing a hidden camera and going up to any random person on the street and saying silly stuff. There was one joke about David Beckham and golden balls or something.

But I loved doing stuff like that and eventually got a gig for a media company, COPA90, to make some videos for the 2014 World Cup in Brazil. They wouldn't let me fly out there to Rio to watch the games, however much I begged. But they gave me a little series of vids to make called Man Versus Football, which involved making content here.

I had to go around the various different nationalities bars in London – so a Portuguese bar when Portugal were playing, a German bar when Germany were on and so on. And there I'd find someone from that country watching the football to have a little chat with.

It was all very ad hoc. I was running around London on my own, there was no producer – I just shot everything myself and had to keep recharging batteries in between meeting people.

The results, I'll be honest, were a little bit hit and miss. The videos bombed and I got trolled online for the first time, people said they were shit.

But the good thing that happened was I kept bumping into this lad along the way – about the same age as me. He was quiet, wore glasses, and said he worked for LBC Radio. He was supposed to be in the bars like me too, collecting quotes from football fans on his dictaphone. But unlike me, this guy Johnny was quite shy. Whereas I was happy to roll up to anyone and make a tit of myself, he seemed reserved and was struggling to get the stuff he needed.

I did a quick recce of the Belgian bar we were in. It was packed – I knew it would be easy to get some quotes and he seemed a little forlorn. 'Here, I'll give you a hand,' I said.

I motored through the crowd in the bar in 10 minutes flat, gave Jonny the content, and didn't think of it again. But the next week I got an email from my agent – Capital FM wanted to meet me. I didn't know it at the time but the young guy I'd helped out in the bar, Johnny, was the son of a broadcasting bigwig at Capital called Richard Park. And he'd sang my praises to his dad. Richard is an incredible man and it's him who I owe my whole radio career to because he got me in and gave me that first shot.

As my mum always says, luck is when preparation meets opportunity. And here – finally – was my opportunity.

MUSIC

I find it weird if I'm doing anything and not listening to music, the silence is too much'

Music is a massive part of who I am. This is hardly surprising – coming from the family I do, with the Godfather I had, and earning my living as a DJ now. Having been in a band myself as a teenager, it's fair to say music has been a constant theme in my life.

I was still at prep school when I made Dad take me to my very first gig to see the American heavy metal band, Slipknot. I was aged about eight, and I was both shit scared and absolutely in awe of these hugely rebellious nine guys on stage. They were all wearing these big scary masks, and had wildly inappropriate song titles like People = Shit. I bloody loved every minute!

But also, thanks to my nan, I'd grown up to the sounds of Frank Sinatra and Elvis, so my tastes are eclectic.

I'm a big believer in the power of music, and how playing different songs has such a different effect on your state of mind and your emotions. Music takes me to a different place every time.

When I listen to songs, I crave that full experience. I'm interested to hear what the artist has been through, what's happened to them to be able to translate a life encounter so effectively into their lyrics and melody.

THE BIG LIST OF MY LIFE

But I'm also intrigued to see what that does to me, how the song makes me feel. I've always believed it's like the artist is triggering a conversation with you. It becomes personal and meaningful. And so it's a really important tool for your own self-reflection, if you like.

Here's some of the things on my playlist…

Music I like to play when I feel sad

Robbie Williams – Millennium
'Stars directing our fate'

Over the last three or four years, I've found myself developing my own personal 'happy song', something I'll play to cheer me up when I need it. A little boost if you like. I first started doing this when I had a girlfriend who lived abroad, and when I was having those horrible pangs of missing her, or when I was feeling generally stressed or overwhelmed with life in any way, putting on Robbie Williams' Millennium seemed to help.

I think that's because I was a kid when I first heard it, I don't remember where I was when it came on, but it brings back feelings of being happy and free from all the worries that inevitably creep up on you as an adult. It's not that the lyrics are all uplifting necessarily, there's quite a cynical line he sings about having 'sarcasm in my eyes' in fact. But it's just that hearing Millennium takes me right back to my childhood, and a time when I didn't feel I was carrying burdens or stress.

Any album by Drake – 6pm in New York
'Some nights I wish I could go back in life. Not to change shit, just to feel a couple things twice'

Of course, there are other times when I don't want to try and cheer myself up. I've found it's actually healthy and cathartic to just have a good old wallow in feeling miserable some days!

At those times, you can't beat sticking on some Drake. The Canadian rapper, singer and songwriter is a genius for moments like this. In fact, there's even a specific term for listening to his albums when you're in this mood – 'Draking', which as a verb is so apt and bloody brilliant!

He basically started a trend for people to listen to sad music and be able to instantly relate to it, and all his woes, as he puts it so much better than you could yourself. Immediately making you feel like you're not the only person feeling like this. That's powerful stuff.

I don't know about you, but I definitely do this little thing where I put on a sad tune and find myself suddenly pretending I'm in the music video for it. So I'll be sitting on a train, headphones on, and looking wistfully off into the distance, with my hand artfully arranged on the window pane. This is how pain looks, people!

If that makes me sound like a melodramatic arse, so be it, because being able to strongly relate to that emotion, and indulgently act it out a bit, does me the world of good. It gives me the chance to reflect on something I've been through from a different perspective. Try it yourself and see!

Music to get me pumped up for a night out

I know this is a thing people do – stick on some tunes while they're getting ready to go out and perhaps have some drinks to get them in the mood. To be honest though, I've never really liked pre-drinks drinks.

THE BIG LIST OF MY LIFE

I don't like to pre-load or get too pumped up because a lot of my nights peak too early if I go down that route as I get tired! So I tried to leave listening to things as last minute as possible, so that I can enjoy the music that I want to listen to at the party I'm actually going to – if that makes sense?

Grime music
Headie One/Stormzy/Central Cee

I love listening to something grimy if I want a bit of adrenaline – a bit of garage, a bit of jungle, a bit of hip hop – I love that energy. But it always has to be the UK genre, I like to hear British voices rapping.

I'm weirdly patriotic about grime because I love the fact we've got artists from these places in the UK where they don't necessarily get a lot of attention, but where you've got these incredible pockets of talent dotted around everywhere and I think that's really something to admire. Some of these kids have come from shit areas, with few opportunities, and they've made some great songs. The energy is so raw.

I've never been able to just sit and listen to house music. I don't like it. Instead I prefer relating to lyrics and learning about people, and being able to listen to their story. As a kid, I was so obsessed with Eminem because it felt like a proper conversation that I could reflect on.

Music to inspire me

Spandau Ballet – The Pride
'Just leave me with the pride that I worked for/
Now they've taken the reason away'

If I'm in a sad mood, or feeling like I need to be inspired, I sometimes listen to a song my Uncle Gary wrote for Spandau Ballet called The Pride.

It's all about his father, my grandad Frank, being made redundant from the printing business. It was a tough time for their family, they were worried about money.

Remembering Grandad makes me proud though. After he lost his job, because all the new technology came along, he didn't sneer and become cynical about the modern world. He actively embraced it. He was the first person to get a computer and a webcam so that he could Skype us. I love that attitude.

Music that gives me a sense of calm

Frank Ocean – Nikes
'Acid on me like the rain / Weed crumbles in the glitter'

Some people might go for ballads, acoustic or even whale music when they want to switch off. Whatever floats your boats. But if I don't want to have any brain distractions I personally find it soothing to listen to rap.

It's the lyrics that do it for me – coming all at once in a big rush. Those lyrics just jump out at you. I always had a knack for learning them quickly and being able to get them out because when I was a kid, my dad used to teach me how to remember lines for the school play.

He explained that it's like having a dominoes effect in your head – once you've mastered the first bit, the next bit will come, and then the next bit and the next bit. I find it's the same thing with rap, the method works and I like using it, almost like a weird tic or scratch that I like exercising.

THE BIG LIST OF MY LIFE

Being able to rap and knowing you've nailed the lyrics can feel hugely satisfying.

So listening to songs like that can be a great distraction – in a way exercise can too – for just taking me out of my head when I need to.

Music for when I'm cooking

 Anything by Ray Charles

I like to go quite old school when I'm in the kitchen – a bit of soul, jazz, blues – is the kind of vibe I seem to want when cooking.

I'm a big fan of the late American singer-songwriter and composer Ray Charles. I love the story behind his music and learning about where those tunes came from, what they mean and what they've done to him. Artists like that always impress me.

I often pick the music appropriate to the food I'm cooking. If I'm making a paella I'll have some Spanish language music on in the background, I'll turn to artists like J Balvin or Bad Bunny. If I'm making some Portuguese dish like a Porco Preto, I'll even throw on some Mas Que Nada.

It's weird but the kitchen is the only place I'll feel comfortable listening to those flowy sorts of old school tunes.

I might even put on a bit of Elvis, which I listened to lots with my nan growing up, in the kitchen.

Nan was obsessed and as I told you, when she wasn't well she said she couldn't wait to die because it would mean she was going up to heaven to marry Elvis, which always makes me smile.

Music for karaoke nights

Robbie Williams – Angels
Harry Styles – Late Night Talking

I love karaoke, we've got one at home for family singalongs, and I've been known to take to the mic with mates too. It appeals to the show-off in me, I guess.

It's brilliant for letting off steam because you can just become someone else entirely in that moment. And the people who are best at karaoke aren't the people that can sing the best. I never judge someone based on their voice, it's always about the performance they give. I like to see some attitude.

So when it comes to choosing tracks, I'll go for something by Robbie Williams or Harry Styles, because they both have that cool kind of bravado you can try and work up while you're belting it out.

When I was in I'm A Celebrity, I had to cover one of Dad's biggest songs, Gold, in karaoke in the Jungle Arms. I got a bit of stick as I didn't know all the words, and I wound Dad up by teasing that I'd actually always preferred Duran Duran. In truth, when I was 17 all that '80s music came back for a bit and I did listen to Spandau Ballet's songs, and enjoyed them. But sorry Dad – they're not on my karaoke wish list!

THE BIG LIST OF MY LIFE

#10

EXERCISE

'How I feel in my body is how I feel in my brain'

Exercise is a crucial part of my life and something that really shores up my mental health.

I've always yo-yoed quite a lot in my weight. That's just how my body is, and I understand that, accept it, and don't beat myself up about that. I try to always ask myself, am I happy? And if I am, then I really try to accept whatever shape I'm in.

But I haven't always had such a healthy attitude towards working out. I over-exercised when I was miserable after the band had failed, and then I had to keep up being thin when I was modelling.

More recently, when I found out I was going into the jungle in 2019, for I'm A Celebrity, I wanted to get in really decent shape for all those inevitable shower scenes.

Before I flew to Australia, for 12 weeks I cut out carbs and did a whole body transformation routine, training every day. I was less busy with work back then, so had the time to do it and enjoyed getting fit.

It was a good experience and I felt in great shape at that time in my life. Though in hindsight, losing so much body fat before I went into the show probably wasn't wise, because I dropped two and half stone in there on jungle food rations

By the time I left the show three weeks later, I remember staring in the mirror looking at myself naked. I looked like an old man, I'd wasted away so much. I was that thin.

When you work in the entertainment industry, I have to be honest, there is a pressure to look a certain way. You've got to look reasonable.

But that's part of the job and I'm happy to take that on my shoulders because I genuinely enjoy working out.

I try to go to the gym four times a week, as well as play football on Wednesday nights. I really get excited about my football night. That's my time to exercise with mates, be sociable, and burn off some pent-up energy with the guys. I think it's useful for many of us to get rid of any aggression that way.

But the gym is my time to be solitary.

In an ideal session, on a Saturday when I have time, I'll do a 40-minute spin class, then an hour of weights, followed by a lovely long sit in a sauna. It's brilliant for clearing my head, then I'll have a bit of a swim.

I love having the time to look after myself in that way, and afterwards it makes me feel so calm, and that sense of peace can last for the rest of the day.

It's one of the best feelings – being tired after exercise – and it helps me sleep better too.

Exercising feels like an achievement, and if you feel like you're achieving something in your day, it's a really simple way to ward off the blues. It's an excellent coping mechanism for dealing with stress.

But it also recharges me. Some days if I've done my radio show in the morning, and then I film The One Show in the evening, I feel like I really need to get to the gym in between as it truly resets me, like a chance to charge your battery.

THE BIG LIST OF MY LIFE

The benefits on body – and brain

When you have depression or anxiety, or just feel low in energy and mood, I know that exercise often feels like the last thing you want to do. We've all been there. But if you can get motivated, it can make a real difference to your mental health.

Some doctors even say that for mild to moderate cases of depression, exercise can be as effective as taking medication.

I do both, because I know what works for me. These are the ways I feel the benefit:

√ My mood improves, thanks to the endorphins and other natural brain chemicals that make me feel good
√ Helps me feel calm for the rest of the day
√ Takes my mind off other worries during the workout – and gives me a better perspective and headspace afterwards
√ It's a coping mechanism and release when I'm feeling frustrated
√ Gives me a little energy boost and wards off fatigue
√ Makes my body feel ready for sleep when it gets to night time
√ Gives me more confidence about my body if I feel in good shape

I know I work out a lot, and not everyone is lucky enough to have that time. But I reckon any exercise is better than none. Start small. Even a 10-minute walk can be a little mood boost, and being outside has proven benefits for mental health too.

Also, it sounds obvious, but try and find something you actually like doing or you won't stick to it! I love the gym and playing football. You might prefer a dance class or boxing lesson. Find the thing that works for you.

FOOD

'My relationship with food is closely tied up with my mental state. If I'm depressed I'll eat terribly'

Have you noticed in recent times there has been a big emphasis on eating well for better gut health? This isn't just a fad. Experts reckon that your gut produces 90 per cent of your serotonin? That's worth bearing in mind when it comes to making food choices, there's lots of advice out there suggesting things like oily fish, fermented foods and those high in fibre may help increase the beneficial bacteria in our gut and improve our brain health.

I'm not claiming to be an expert on nutrition, but I do think that's interesting.

And I know, for me, there's a definite link between what I'm eating and how I'm feeling. My relationship with food is closely tied up with my mental state. If I'm depressed I'll eat terribly, I'll reach for crap and gain weight, which makes me feel lethargic and I get stuck in a cycle. I've learned that getting my diet right can really help me feel better about myself.

When I'm feeling focused on my career, and in control of my life, it feels easier to fuel my body the right way. A lot of the time it's about having structure, to make sure you're eating well. But I know first hand when you're busy and stressed it's so easy for that to go out of the window.

And society adds pressure – you feel like you're a 'good

person' if you're maintaining a healthy diet and a 'bad person' when it's all gone to shit. I try not to beat myself up about food and just try to enjoy it.

It was my mum who did the cooking in our house as a kid. Dad is terrible in the kitchen. I once watched him put peanut butter and tomato ketchup together because he genuinely thought it would make a good pasta sauce. Obviously it was completely rank!

Lots of people say a Sunday roast is their very favourite meal, I'm sure this is more because they associate it with love and being cared for as much as any flavour.

We didn't have Sunday roasts in our house. Mum, Dad and Harley are all veggie, and we were brought up on all sorts of different foods from around the world, like sushi and curries. Mum can do a decent curry but she was never really that much into cooking, she got me and Harley busy in the kitchen as early as she could.

Sometimes this worked to my advantage as a kid, if Mum saw I was struggling to concentrate on a maths project or English spellings she'd let me sit at the kitchen counter instead.

'That's fine, Ro, if you don't want to do homework,' she'd say. 'But you have to do something useful'. So I'd be allowed to sit and help her make dinner. By 13 I was pretty much making my own dinner. It's probably one of the reasons why I love cooking so much now.

Having the time to cook is such a luxury and when I get to do it, I'm a happy boy. There's something very therapeutic and mindful about the whole process of choosing, preparing and seeing it come to life.

As well as the pleasure I get from feeding other people. I've learned that balance is key – and food should be something to savour and enjoy. So I try to make eating a pleasure in life, not something else I can punish myself for.

Here are some of my go-to dishes:

Boring breakfast boy

Everyone at Capital takes the piss out of me because I am the most boring breakfast eater in the world. My favourite morning meal, that I rarely divert from, is porridge mixed with jam and peanut butter.

And I like my porridge the way I like pasta, which is al dente. It looks disgusting I have to admit, it comes out really clumpy, so it must seem like I'm eating paper mache every day.

The only times I deviate is when I sometimes have oatmeal, or yoghurt or bran flakes. Yes, I know I am weird.

Anything that comes with broccoli

Weirdly, until I was three, all I wanted to eat was broccoli, for breakfast, lunch and dinner. Healthy – yes. But very strange. It's still my all-time favourite vegetable.

Veggie sausage sandwiches after footy

When I'd come home freezing from playing football in the rain as a kid, Mum would make me go in the bath. I can still remember the stinging feel of going from cold to hot. Then I'd come downstairs and Mum made veggie sausage sandwiches. That's comfort food for me.

I mainly grew up on veggie food, until I asked Mum if I could eat meat, it was only Harley that wanted to be like them.

THE BIG LIST OF MY LIFE

Spaghetti Bolognese

Everyone seems to believe that they themselves make the best Bolognese sauce, don't they? Myself included! And whether making veggie or meat I always use my mum's secret trick of adding some ketchup in there. It definitely makes it taste better.

Curries 🌶🌶🌶

Indian food was a big staple in our house and my all-time favourite meal with family and with friends is still curry. And I cook a mean one myself. That's my go-to for feeding friends.

Growing up, there was a curry house in Highgate called Kipling's where we spent many family meals. Every time I pass it I can still remember the smell and taste of the poppadoms, the mango chutney, the korma or tikka masala.

I get weirdly patriotic sometimes, and see Chicken Tikka Masala as a real British dish these days.

I wouldn't eat a curry alone, for me the whole joy is sitting and sharing them with friends and feeling together. That's the best vibe for Indian food.

Pizza (no pineapple!)

Pizza is always king – whether it's for celebrating or comfort, it's a regular part of my diet. But one thing I am very firm on – pineapple has NO place on a pizza.

Give me pizza over chocolate any day. Dad worried as a kid because I seemed to eat vast quantities all the time. 'It's not good for you, Ro, it's the worst thing you can eat,' he'd complain. But that only made me want it more.

A nice, simple chicken and chips

Joe and I would be regulars at Nando's. We'd set the world to rights and talk about everything going on in our lives and at work over half a chicken and chips. Sometimes the simple things really are the best.

Salty popcorn (no sweet stuff)

If I'm at the cinema, I'm the guy ordering a bucket of straight salty popcorn. No mixing with the sweet stuff for me. I've been intrigued by people's taste buds, everyone has an order they like, and mine is savoury, sweet, and then back to savoury.

But I think that's just being called greedy! Don't get me wrong, I've got a sweet tooth too. I am my dad's son, after all. Dad eats an insane amount of chocolate. He even wakes up in the middle of the night and the first thing he thinks about is going downstairs into the kitchen and eating chocolate out of the fridge. He tries to do it without my mum knowing, and will lie to her when she's caught him out.

What I cook to impress

I don't have one specific meal I cook for a date, because I always like to cater for whatever that person enjoys eating most. Whether it's a truffle risotto or burrata side salad, I'll give it a go.

I love finding out what someone likes, and if I've never made it before, even better.

I dated an Argentinian girl for a little bit and we would make Argentinian food and sizzle steak together, and that was fantastic.

THE BIG LIST OF MY LIFE

One time I had promised to cook for a girl coming over and I was totally chockablock at work. I really wanted to impress her and thought I had all the ingredients ready and the oven on.

Then I realised a key ingredient was an onion – which I had failed to get.

I couldn't leave the house as I'm funny about going out with the oven on, and I was in the middle of it all, so I basically had to Deliveroo a single onion. Because of the delivery fee it cost me £7, and I did feel a bit upper-class as this geezer arrived and handed over the lone, unbagged onion.

It was a particularly bougie moment I admit, and I ended up with people having a go at me for that as it made it into the papers.

I always tell myself that when I stop doing the breakfast show and lead a less crazy life, I'll really enjoy cooking a lot more. It's a real fantasy for me to have a wife and kids one day and be able to spend my evenings making their meals and giving them love and nurture that way.

SLEEP

'It was a girl I was dating who first pointed out to me that during the night I stopped breathing. She noticed that I stopped breathing for 10, then 15, then 20 seconds'

There's a close link between sleep and mental health. And if you're not getting enough of it, then it does start messing with your head. Low mood, irritability and lack of concentration are all problems. Especially if you're already at risk of depression or anxiety, a bad night's sleep – or many nights of bad sleep – is not good news as it escalates all that and affects your emotions.

As a kid I was always trying to stay up late. I'd have the telly on with one ear listening out for my dad, and if I heard him stomp across the hallway I'd race to turn off the TV and dive back into bed pretending to be asleep so he wouldn't tell me off.

Until I was about eight, I'd always want to sleep in my sister's bed, which was no doubt annoying for her. But then as a teenager, of course I found I could lie in all day if I was allowed to.

I've always had the ability to shut my eyes and have a nap anywhere. When I worked in the gym I'd even take myself off to a cupboard in my lunch break and curl up in there for a quick snooze.

But when you work in breakfast radio, getting up at the

crack of dawn every day doesn't feel healthy. My alarm is set before 5am and I try to get into bed before 11pm. I reckon I run on about five-and-a-half hours a night, which isn't enough. And I think I'm the only breakfast presenter in history who doesn't drink coffee to power me through.

I like to try to catch up with sleep on my holidays, but that always makes me feel bad, like going on holiday with me will be the most boring time ever as I'll be in bed half the day.

For years I've suffered from sleep deprivation, where the fatigue has often felt totally debilitating, like being in a constant fog and having no energy. I blamed my intense work schedule, and I even thought I might have narcolepsy, which is a brain condition that causes people to suddenly fall asleep. I could literally be mid-conversation and I'd be falling asleep and starting to snore! It was very strange.

I realised it couldn't just be my work hours because all my colleagues at the station were coping just fine. I found myself looking around and being jealous of everyone else, as they went off to have a nice afternoon after work and all I could think of was when I could fall asleep next. I wanted to be out living my life too, instead I became obsessed with sleep. What the fuck was wrong with me? I had my iron levels tested and that was fine.

Recently, I saw a doctor and was diagnosed with sleep apnoea, which is when your breathing stops and starts when you're asleep. I've got the most common kind of the condition, which is obstructive sleep apnoea (OSA), which means that the muscles of my throat can relax and block my airways during my sleep.

It also means I can snore loudly – there ain't nothing sexy about it, I can tell you!

According to the NHS, here are the symptoms:

- Breathing stopping and starting
- Making gasping, snorting or choking noises
- Waking up a lot
- Loud snoring

It also means that when you're awake you feel generally knackered, you struggle to concentrate, and can feel moody and headachey. Nice.

It was a girl I was dating who first pointed out to me that during the night I stopped breathing. I'm a single guy, but had been dating and she'd stayed over a few times. She noticed that I stopped breathing for 10, then 15, then 20 seconds. It put me in a panic and when I had it checked out, the doctor confirmed the sleep apnoea. It's been rubbish, to be honest.

I'm being monitored, but it means that at night time I have to wear an oxygen mask to bed. It doesn't exactly make me the most romantic or sexiest bed mate, me lying there doing my best Darth Vader impression. I've started joking that my love life will look like a niche Channel 5 documentary.

I'm fine really, it's not life threatening, but it's a bit embarrassing sleeping with the mask, and a tab on my finger, plus something monitoring my neck. But it's reassuring the docs are keeping an eye on it.

I'm hoping one day I'll be able to get the right surgery on my tonsils and back of throat to be able to sort it out.

In an ideal world I'd be running on seven hours' shut-eye a night. I see it like a battery on your phone and it recharges you and sets you up for the day. And hopefully I'll get there.

THE BIG LIST OF MY LIFE

MATES

***'The guys who don't think they have any
problems and don't need to talk can be the ones
who end up in the biggest trouble actually'***

Lovers come and go but friendships never end. I'm sure the Spice Girls had some wise words along those lines. And hopefully your mates are there through thick and thin. My best ones are Charlie and Matt, who've both known me since I was six.

Matt and Charlie were like the real cool kids at the school and the best at football. Matt even went on to play professionally for Slough. Charlie's dad was the football coach, we really ended up forming a really close kind of bond. Charlie moved to the same secondary school as me. Matt went somewhere different. But the three of us remained ridiculously close.

When we were around 12, Charlie's mum got diagnosed with breast cancer. She slowly deteriorated, and then sadly, she passed away. We were just kids. He was so calm about it at the time, but clearly dealt with his pain a lot in silence behind the scenes. It wasn't until years later that we really talked about it.

Charlie's the first person I ever opened up to about mental health. And I was the first person to hear about his.

I remember sitting in the car with him when we were 17. I'd been taking my tablets for two years and he was the first friend I told.

Afterwards, he too suddenly opened up fully about his anxieties, panic attacks, his fear of death and all these types of things. We chatted and later he went for CBT therapy, which really helped.

Being able to talk frankly like that gave me a buddy system – which is what all young men need. And this is something we highlight in Joe's Buddy Line, which I'll tell you more about later. Once I'd spoken truthfully to Charlie that day, I then had that one person who was outside of my family who I could go to after having a shit day.

It's so good to have that. It's something that I've always pushed to guys, even having just one friend who can be there for you.

Matt is someone on the other end of the spectrum, Matt is someone who has never obviously had mental health issues. He's the loudest, most confident, outrageously competent guy. But the more I've learned about suicide I've realised that people like him, the Matts of this world, are still at risk.

The guys who don't think they have any problems and don't need to talk can be the ones who end up in the biggest trouble actually.

As well as being a pillar of strength and support for me, Matt can take the piss like no one else. He has me in his phone as 'Roman Kemp Z' – for Z-list.

He rather rudely changes the letter up or down depending on how my career is going. After I'm A Celeb I got to J — but he demoted me when I did a TV show called Bromans. I think I'm back up to the dizzying height of Roman Kemp G now. Cheeky fucker.

It's Matt and Charlie who keep me level-headed and remind me of my glory days making Pitch Invasion TV.

We're very close but very different characters. Charlie's my sensible friend, Matt's my crazy friend. Charlie's the first at any party, Matt's always the last standing, and I suppose I sit somewhere in the middle.

They're like a married couple. They still share a flat in Camberwell and remain my stabilising force in life. They keep me grounded and I couldn't be without them. I'm very lucky.

Famous pals – name-dropping time

I'm very fortunate with the people that I've been able to claim as friends in this oh-so-fickle industry.

Ed Sheeran

Ed is such a decent guy and someone I'll turn to for advice about my career. For someone with that unbelievable level of success he's the most down-to-earth person you can imagine. You can't find any fault with Ed. He's such a big supporter of his mates as well as being a real talent. He's a dad now, he has his baby and his wife to focus on. And he's very sorted. But I've had some fun nights drinking wine with him over the years.

Harry Styles

For me, Harry has now reached superstar status, he's the next David Bowie or Mick Jagger I reckon. He'll have staying power.

But what I love doing best with Harry is playing football in the park. Niall Horan plays too, then we'll get some food in Camden. None of this VIP shit. Harry's a very grounded guy.

I was there interviewing Harry when he released his first

song so I feel like I've been there for his whole journey. We're the same age and in the same industry, so we share a lot in common.

Lewis Capaldi

Lewis is a top bloke – but a bit of a liability in my life. Every time he is in town and wants to go out I will be like, 'Oh, go on then.' And it sometimes gets messy. At one point I'd get a drunken FaceTime call from him at least once a week at about 4am.

But he's such a great guy. Like Ed, he doesn't let his success change him. Our favourite nights out together are just in a local 'old man' pub.

Justin Bieber

I haven't spoken to Justin in a while now, but I've had some fun times with him. He's a lot more serious and focused now, but when he first came to London around his Purpose album (in 2015) he was out every night for three weeks!

He came on to the show, we chatted and decided to go out to a party. Every girl in the room was looking at him, it was a different world.

THE BIG LIST OF MY LIFE

MONEY

***'My parents' relationship with cash made them
very anxious. And that trickled down to me'***

Everyone knows the joke that money doesn't buy you happiness – but it sure does help.

What is certainly no laughing matter is that people with mental health problems are three-and-a-half times as likely to be in problem debt.

Our relationships with our finances can be complex, and money woes can be devastating. Joe often talked about money and was always dreaming up the next way to make his fortune. In the aftermath of his death I felt a huge amount of guilt, about many things actually, but one was about money. As a presenter I was paid more than him as a producer. Is that right or fair? Probably not. It's the way it works, but living with that thought isn't easy.

I know full well how privileged I am because money problems don't keep me awake at night.

I can only be honest about my own attitude to money – and if you think it's annoying me sitting here with my nice job and life, then I'm sorry. Please feel free to turn the page as I fully realise I could come across as a privileged arsehole…

People think that if you're on telly, you are automatically rich. I can tell you that's not true. I've always been aware of money and not taken it for granted. I have money, I earn a good wage, but I'm savvy and know not to waste it.

My parents' relationship with cash made them very anxious. And that definitely trickled down to me.

But it also taught me early on that I needed to get better educated about my finances.

Dad always talked about them being 'cheque to cheque' people. Because that's how you live in our industry. You're not paid the same amount monthly. As a freelancer it could be tempting to get paid and think that's yours for spending. Then later realise, 'shit, I've got to pay tax on it'. Or this or that. Hidden things you don't cater for. Or you might not work for a few months.

As soon as I tell Mum and Dad I've got a job, they always want to know how much I'm being paid and they warn me, 'Make sure you put that away safely.'

If I buy a new pair of shoes, the first question Mum will ask is, 'How much did they cost?' They're terrified I'll have money woes and all the stress they bring.

I don't like spending money for the sake of it. For being flash. We ain't those types of people.

My dad came from a home where he lived with three other families – my cousins, my aunties, the whole extended family was squashed up in there. There was a toilet outside and an air raid shelter in the yard.

Before Dad and Uncle Gary made their name in the band, and some decent cash, the surname 'Kemp' was a pauper name. When we were on a TV show called DNA Journey, Dad and I learned all about our past relatives. Dad's granny, Eta, was forced into the workhouses aged just 13. (I've got her name tattooed on my arm too.)

THE BIG LIST OF MY LIFE

Dad's mum Eileen was a dinner lady. And Dad's dad, Frank, worked in the printing business. When he was made redundant because of all the new technology, Dad remembers his mum crying one day in the kitchen because she was so scared she wouldn't have food to feed her kids. She was trying to make a pie, but could only afford the potato, not the meat.

My mum grew up in a small council house too.

My parents had to spend their whole life savings – the money from their music careers – on expensive medical treatment for Dad's tumour in America because it wasn't available here. We're talking millions of pounds, gone in the space of a few years.

They faced bankruptcy and we downsized to a smaller house and lost the nice Jeep with the electric windows. Suddenly we were driving around in a knackered old car with windows that kept sticking as you rolled them down manually. But I'm not moaning – I appreciate that's a real first-world problem.

I remember being in awe of Harley getting her first Saturday job aged 13 and feeling under pressure to do the same.

When I started earning money, when I joined the band and then later got into radio, Mum and my dad were so scared of me wasting it.

Given their upbringings, and losing their savings, it's hardly surprising Mum and Dad are anxious about cash. They always instil in me the need for savings, to cope with an emergency situation like they faced. You never know what's around the corner, they warn me. They're so up on all the penny-pinching tips, it was like living with money saving expert Martin Lewis!

But as I've become an adult, it's me in the end who taught them about the bigger stuff – mortgages, interest rates, the importance of making wills and taking out insurance. I want them to feel financially secure. When Harley recently bought a house it wasn't Mum and Dad she rang for advice, it was me she was on the phone to constantly.

When I was given the breakfast slot at Capital, I was over the moon. The salary was five times higher than what I'd been on before. But I was also really scared I wasn't worth it and wouldn't be up to it.

I actually told the bosses that yes please, I wanted the job but could they keep my money the same as I was already on for the first year. I didn't want that pressure and basically gave them an out. I said, 'Pay me the same money – and I'll come back for that money in a year's time if I've done a good job.'

Joe thought I was mad, and he happily took his pay rise. But I thought that was fair and right, I wanted to hold up my end of the bargain.

Dad is proud of me for finding a career I love, but I think he would have been equally proud so long as I'd got off my arse and found a job that earned me any living. He doesn't care about fame or riches at all.

When I bought my first flat I had to ask Dad if I could borrow some cash – there were all these extras I needed towards stamp duty and the deposit. It was tens of thousands, and Dad helped me out. But he also said he needed it back in six weeks. So I made sure I took on extra work. Some jobs I didn't necessarily want to do and I paid it back in full.

When I first started earning and getting the hang of doing my own taxes, I found it stressful to be confronted with a tax bill. Most of my friends are taxed at source so I didn't have people to talk to about it. But it was a learning experience, I was growing up, and I know what I'm doing now.

So money doesn't keep me awake at night. And that's because I've worked hard and genned up on managing it properly. I have savings I put aside and I'm pretty frugal. When I first started earning some money, I used to buy so many clothes thinking it was cool to hit Selfridges and get the latest Balenciaga or designer stuff like that.

But as I've got older I've developed more sense. What's worth spending on and what isn't? It's not worth spending £350 on a T-shirt. But a grand on a decent suit you'll wear again and again? Yes, I'd see that as an investment in myself. And if it helps you feel pulled together and smart, and you're fortunate to have the funds, it's worth it.

####

> **'Mum sent me a photo on the family WhatsApp of refugees in Africa wearing my smartest tuxedo shoes! I said 'Mum – I love those shoes!"**

####

Mum makes me have a regular clearout of my clothes and give what I don't need to charity. She literally comes over to my house, sometimes lets herself in, and takes away stuff she thinks I don't need and someone else might benefit from.

She sent me a photo on the family WhatsApp of refugees in Africa wearing my smartest tuxedo shoes! I said 'Mum – I love those shoes!'

The next picture she shared was of a bloke proudly wearing my football boots. Literally I'd only been playing in them the week before.

'Oh you don't need them,' she replies. 'Other people have

less than you.' She's absolutely right, and that's why I love her and she makes me laugh.

The one thing that I do spend money on is holidays. And I don't feel guilty about that. They're important to me, I know I work hard and I want to enjoy that time off.

If I'm earning more than mates, I'm happy to pay them to come. I know they are keen to do the same back and worry if they can't. But I don't care at all. What's the point otherwise?

I've already planned for when I have kids – I'll treat them to the holidays and spoil them that way, but for everything else they'll have to sort themselves out.

I love my job and want to do well. But I always dream of retiring, not thinking about money, and living a simple life.

THE BIG LIST OF MY LIFE

TATTOOS

'Niall Horan from One Direction tattooed 'Nice to melt ya' on my foot. It was supposed to say the name of his new single, 'Nice To Meet Ya'. Cheers for that, Niall'

Getting tattoos has become a regular part of my life.

At important times, or if something has happened that matters to me, I go to the shop and get one. It's like an urge I feel in moments of stress.

There's a term that people use called 'getting blasted'. That's when they get one tattoo, and then they want another one. And another one.

Tattoo artists recognise that, they see it all the time. There's a running joke within tattoo parlours where the artists can always tell if someone's just broken up with a partner, or if they're going through something heavy, because all of a sudden they're in the tattoo shop every week!

Tattoo artists are great listeners, I find. I've spent lots of time where I've sat down and just chatted to them about stuff that's going on in my life. They've seen it all before and I don't feel judged.

The main reason I started getting inked was because my Grandad Henry, my mum's dad, developed dementia in later life. I started wondering whether I might go the same way one day. So by having important people, and animals I love inked onto my body, I hope that one day, when I'm an old man, I'll still be able to remember the things that mattered most in my life.

I honestly couldn't tell you how many I have now – too many to count! – but here are some of the more important ones for me:

I've got an anchor and a large eagle across my torso: Dad's dad signed up to the Navy when he was young – mainly because back then they were offering free tattoos as an incentive! So on one of his forearms he had an anchor. I was fascinated as a kid and loved touching it.

The eagle is just because they're amazing. I love animals and I'm fascinated by them. I've also got a great white shark on the back of my arm. I like remembering that we share this planet, it's not just ours. I wanted to pay respect to these magnificent creatures we inhabit this earth with.

I've got the steam train that my great-grandad used to drive for the King of Egypt (yes, how ridiculous): And one of the last cards my nan – my mum's mother – ever wrote to me was signed off 'lots of love'. So I've got that in her handwriting on my rib cage. I've got all the important women in my life somewhere too – both grandmothers, a great-grandmother, my mum and sister.

On my back I've got the hand of Fatima, which is like an ancient protection symbol often seen in Judaism or Islam: I'm not tied to any religion but I liked the symbol, and my dad and sister have the same thing so Harley encouraged me to have it. I felt like it I wanted to make it more personal, and as it's a female protection sign, I got my mum to draw an outline around her hand and took a picture of her eye and used that. I love the idea of my own kids one day being able to hold their hands against Mum's. I've got a moon crescent in that same tattoo to represent Harley too.

I've got a tattoo of a dove on my leg in honour of Joe: He had the same tattoo in the same place. And I'd take the piss out of it and tell him it looked like a shit pigeon, not a dove. Now I boast the exact same one, which makes me think of him and also makes me smile.

I've also got some slightly dubious tattoos my mum isn't keen on…. Ed Sheeran badly tattooed 'Ed woz ere 2k7 x' on my leg live on air for charity. Later, I had a female fan of Ed's come up to me and offer £20k if I'd take the skin off my leg and put it in formaldehyde. Funnily enough, I said no.

Plus Niall Horan from One Direction tattooed 'Nice to melt ya' on my foot. It was supposed to say the name of his new single, 'Nice To Meet Ya'. Cheers for that, Niall. He did generously donate £5,000 to charity afterwards though.

I haven't got any tattoos of any ex-girlfriends, and if a girl hated my tattoos then I'm sorry, they're staying put! I'd never get rid of them.

Mum generally rolls her eyes every time I get a new one and says, 'Please don't get any more, Ro!'

But I've no plans to stop.

#16

DRINK AND DRUGS

'I found it a very sobering thought, this statistic that half of people with a mental illness are likely to abuse booze and drugs'

After a hard day at work, loads of people reach for a drink as a quick way to relax. I know it might make you feel better initially, but drinking alcohol regularly can actually make stress and anxiety worse. Similarly, we might think booze helps us to be more sociable. It lowers inhibitions, making us feel confident. But once the effects of the drink wear off – you can definitely be left feeling more anxious and paranoid than you did before.

I don't want to lecture anyone about how they should live their lives – I'm not Mr Perfect.

But the facts about booze and the negative impact it has on our mental health can't be ignored, and nor should it be underestimated. Drink is one of the biggest factors affecting young male mental health.

When I was researching it, I came across Richie Perera, who founded Mental Health and Life, an organisation aimed at raising awareness of mental health in the UK. He's also written a book called Managing People In The New Normal*. He has a really useful way of thinking and talking about mental health, which he calls the continuum of mental health.

We all exist somewhere on the mental health continuum

in one of the four quadrants and can move around it yearly, monthly and even daily.

This was a helpful concept – to see that how we feel about our mental health is a constantly changing landscape. It can stop you labelling yourself as someone with 'poor' or 'good' mental health and actually be more mindful in paying attention to how you're really doing at this point in time. Not last year, not next year if your dreams come true. But NOW.

The mental health continuum helps us to understand that as long as we are living and breathing, mental ill-health is a given due to the risk factors we are all faced with in general life. What are these risk factors?

Well, risk factors for mental ill-health can range from drug and substance abuse, to trauma as an adult or a child, to financial hardships and all the way to long-term stress. According to Richie, that is far from an exhaustive list. He believes it is not possible to have the most basic understanding of mental health awareness without an understanding of this mental health continuum.

The foundation of mental health awareness is what he calls the 'holy quad-trinity' of wellbeing:

- Diet – because your gut produces 90 per cent of your serotonin which is directly connected to your mood, memory, sleep, sexual function and bone health to name a few.

- Exercise – because it is essential for overall health and experts are now recognising that it can work as well as antidepressants for some people.

- Sleep – Richie insists eight hours of solid sleep is needed for both the body and mind to repair, regenerate and rejuvenate every single day. (This might be a stretch for many of us, I appreciate.)

- Digitally detoxing – the average person in the UK spends 34 years staring at screens! Richie says living on screens is the opposite of our human nature and the needs and wants of our mental and physical health. I can certainly see the point in this argument.

Talking about alcohol and substance abuse, Richie says: 'Its impact on mental health and wellbeing are playing havoc with people's lives due to the way they are embedded in British culture'. I was told the UK spent an astonishing £26 billion on alcohol in 2020. And we are saying 'yes' to drugs like never before. Londoners consume more cocaine on a daily basis than people living in Barcelona, Berlin and Amsterdam combined. In fact, drink and drug abuse is so rife here in the UK, traces of cocaine were found in 11 out of 12 toilets at Parliament.

Every week, 28 per cent of men and 25 per cent of women binge drink every week. It is no wonder that 50 per cent of people with a mental illness have problems with alcohol and substance misuse. I found it a very sobering thought, this statistic that half of people with a mental illness are likely to abuse booze and drugs. As Richie says, alcohol really is embedded in our culture here in Britain.

My first introduction to alcohol was when my dad and my grandad took me to the football when I was a kid and I used to make smiley faces in the froth of my dad's Guinness. I tried a sip and thought it was revolting. My first experience of getting pissed was very early, aged 11 years old, at a mate's house in Chorleywood.

We had a friend who seemed to have a free house all the time, with no adults around, and which also seemed to be filled with an endless supply of Smirnoff Ice, WKDs, and all those sweet alcohol-pop drinks marketed at teenagers. We even seemed to think J20s, the fruit juice, contained alcohol at one point. Clueless.

We had some weird ideas about how you got drunk in those days. My mate Charlie opened a tin of lager, something very weak like a Foster's, and we all gingerly took a swig and passed it round the room, thinking this was what grown-up drinkers did. It tasted gross. But we all pretended it was good. I imagine most of us thought it was disgusting initially – and yet the majority of us carried on! But with drinking, as Richie says, it's so ingrained in our make-up that most of us push through those early instincts not to like it and force ourselves to continue.

In many ways I am fortunate that drinking has never been a massive part of my life. The only time I was ever sick from drinking was when I went on a football school trip to Cyprus aged 14, and all the sixth-form lads made me drink an entire bottle of Sambuca.

But honestly I've never been sick through booze since, nor have I ever blacked out. I love my job more than any alcohol, and I never want to be hungover on radio, so I never drink at all during the week. And the idea of daytime drinking never appeals. These are my rules and I'm sticking to them. It's served me well.

Of course, I'm not perfect. I'm a young guy living in London and getting drunk on the weekends with mates is part of that. But I also have to be honest about the effects it has on me. I know when I'm hungover I'm in a horrible place. All my bad thoughts are there right in my face. That's gotten worse as I've gotten older. Not just because you feel more physical effects the morning after, but because you have more pressures in life generally. And those do come out after we drink.

My anxiety is absolutely through the roof the day after I've been drinking. I start worrying about things that I should never worry about, and all the things that I perhaps should worry about send me into extreme panic! I have to always try and surround myself with the right people the next day because I don't want to be alone.

The fact I know how bad drinking can make me feel the next day massively puts me off. I know what it's like if you're unhappy, you can feel like you have to be out a lot, and drinking helps in that moment to forget all your worries. I've got friends who do this. And now I've become the sensible one at times, who tries to remind them how much shitter they'll feel the next day. And how if you drink again to make yourself feel better, you're suddenly stuck in this awful cycle.

Another thing that's done me a favour I think is that my parents aren't massive drinkers. I wasn't brought up with much alcohol around the house. And now if we go out for a family meal I'll order a Diet Coke most of the time and Dad will follow suit. We're all warned of the dangers of drugs – but in my opinion alcohol is the worst of them all and yet it's so readily available. I do have to be mindful about drinking.

As for smoking... I tried my first cigarette in that friend's kitchen too, around the age of 11, with my friend Will. It was something rank like Benson & Hedges, no doubt nicked from a packet belonging to someone's parents. Lighting it up felt the height of sophistication. But as soon as I took that first drag and inhaled, I instantly wanted to vomit. What a revolting taste! It was gross.

Growing up, I'd also seen my mum's mum, my nan Maggie, on a nebulizer for most of my life. I'd learned how to fill it up for her and put it on her face. She'd grown up as part of that generation of people who didn't know the risks of smoking, so she'd merrily puffed away, then it became a habit she couldn't quit, and for as long as I could remember, she had horrendous lung problems as a result. So my nan, plus that first unpleasant experience of having a cigarette, did a wonderful job of putting me off smoking for good.

And then there's drugs. Unfortunately it's a rite of passage for many young people to dabble in weed and stuff when they're a teenager. Hey, even the former President of the United States of America, Bill Clinton, admitted to having a little toke and got himself all in a PR tangle… (although he didn't inhale, right? Ha ha.)

Without getting heavy, the bottom line is the obvious fact that drugs are illegal. So you could risk getting a criminal record which could lose you your job, even your liberty. No one wants that, right?! But even after that, there's plenty we need to be aware of – they're just not good for mental health. More than that in fact, drug abuse is one of the leading causes of mental ill-health these days. So I'm never gonna come out in support of them.

I imagine drugs are part of a young person's rebellion? But with my parents, there wasn't that much to rebel against. Mum might have asked me, 'You're not getting drunk are you?' I'd say, 'Of course not!' (When of course I was.)

She was terrified I might become a 'dope smoker' as she called it. But I've always been a relatively sensible person in this area. Dad has never lectured me or Harley and said 'don't take this' or 'don't do that'. And Mum has always believed that if you ban things and make them forbidden to young people, then the desire to do it becomes even stronger. There's something to be said for this kind of reverse psychology. If they had banned me from anything they probably know I would do the opposite.

When I was in the band, we often stayed with this guy – someone from the record label who we'd go and write music with. He was about 40 and was pretty 'out there' – he used to inject himself with snake venom. Seriously. He said it was for medicinal reasons, but watching him slice his arm open with a razor blade and then rub in this snake venom was quite a reality check! And it made me shit-scared of that whole murky scene.

I plan to tell my own kids one day not to do things like drink or take drugs, but I'm aware there are certain things you're just gonna try because you can and you wanna look cool. But it's worth remembering how it's the very opposite of cool when you feel broken inside the next day.

I am not claiming to be an expert and I'm not the drink and drug police, but there are widely proven facts we need to remember:

Facts we can't ignore about booze

How alcohol affects our brains: The chemical changes in your brain can mean more negative feelings – like anxiety, depression, anger or aggression – start to take over. This is because alcohol affects the neurotransmitters in your brain. These are chemicals that send messages from one nerve in your brain to another –

and alcohol stops them from working correctly. Alcohol affects your brain chemistry – fact. Signs that alcohol is harming your mental health include:

- Finding it hard to sleep after drinking
- Having a low mood
- Feeling tired and hungover regularly
- Feeling worried and anxious in places and with people that you wouldn't normally have any worries about

Tips to cut down alcohol:

- Stay within the low-risk guidelines – this means not drinking more than 14 units of alcohol a week spread out over three days or more
- Don't drink on an empty stomach
- Alternate soft drinks and alcoholic ones
- Have several 'dry' days a week
- Switch to lower strength or alcohol-free drinks
- Keep a diary of your drinking and check in with it every few weeks to track how you're doing*.

I hope that all didn't sound like a lecture. Like I say, I'm no expert and far from perfect, but we need to take care of ourselves. Make sure you check out the info at the end of the book if you need help with anything to do with drink and drugs guys…

*(SOURCES:https://www.betterhealth.vic.gov.au/health/healthyliving/How-drugs-affectyour-body AND https://www.bupa.co.uk/newsroom/ourviews/alcohol-and-mental-health AND https://alcoholchange.org.uk/alcohol-facts/fact-sheets/alcohol-and-mental-health)

#17

MY PHONE

'I think it's too easy to blame social media sometimes, schools are quick to say kids' mental health is all down to social media use, when often it's actually to do with a previous trauma or what's going on at home'

We all know the mental health benefits of a digital detox, but how many of us actually step away from our mobiles and regularly do it? Hands down, one of the best things about being in the jungle was being forcibly parted from my phone.

It's hard to resist scrolling. But when that wasn't an option, I realised I felt much lighter. And I started questioning how much my phone, and using social media, actually enriches my life. Not a lot, I concluded.

In fact, when the producers gave me the phone back, I honestly didn't want it. I was so scared of it, I daren't even turn it on for three weeks!

I've had conversations with my mate Ed Sheeran about this, because we both get stressed out by our phones. He now gets people to email him instead. I can see the benefit of putting that little bit of distance in place. Every time Ed sees me he says, 'You've just got to get rid of the phone, mate!'

I do fantasise about it.

We're all familiar with phone stress...

- Analysing blue ticks on WhatsApp?!
- Being left on 'read'?!
- The constant pinging from big group chats?!

We all have to navigate our own boundaries – and I'm still working on mine.

Same with social media. I love it and loathe it at times.

We're all guilty of scrolling through Instagram and seeing someone moaning about life being so tough. And then you look at all their Ferraris and fancy holidays and you think, 'Yeah right, mate,' and roll your eyes. I know I have. I'm as guilty as anyone else of seeing what someone like Brooklyn Beckham is up to, and assuming a) he got there purely because of who his dad is, and b) assuming they have a charmed, woe-free existence.

I know I should know better, but that whole set-up of social media makes us compare ourselves to each other, and it's worth remembering – it's not real!

Everyone looks like they're having the best time of their life on there and you start feeling like you're coming up short. Everyone becomes someone else on social media. Whether it's a 'better' version or a 'funnier' version, it's never quite that real person.

People say to me, 'Oh you're not who I thought you'd be from social media,' and leave you feeling like you're a disappointment in real life. But it also starts you wondering – well, who am I then?

It goes back to this constant inner conflict I have about the professional front and how I feel inside. I feel it's part of my job to post the things I've been up to, it's expected, and I get that.

But what I post on Instagram is Roman Kemp – it's not really me, Ro.

I stopped posting pics of the guests I had on the show because it felt like everyone would think I had this amazing life and was best mates with all these celebrities. That isn't true, and I hated that it made me look very 'beggy' – desperate for validation and chasing likes. So I stopped doing that.

At the end of the day I treat Instagram like a business tool, I'm quite open about that, I do adverts and things. I share a few private pics but not many. I know some people in our industry have a work account and then a private account – but I can't be arsed with that. If I want to show someone who matters to me what I'm up to, then I'll just pick up the phone and tell them!

I think it's too easy to blame social media sometimes, schools are quick to say kids' mental health is all down to social media use, when often it's actually to do with a previous trauma or what's going on at home. Social media can provide a place where kids get bullied these days. But that's the way society is going. There's going to be a different platform or different method for doing that every two months.

I've tried imposing rules about limiting my phone use, and not having it in the bedroom, but at the end of the day I also can't resist having a scroll through football things before I go to sleep.

What I don't like

Selfies

I hate having my photo taken, I do sometimes post selfies but, quite honestly, they make me cringe. I don't like going through my Instagram and seeing old pictures of myself because I will then compare it with how I am now. Did I look better then? Did I feel better? Or find myself wishing I could go back and be at that time again. It's just not healthy.

Instagram couples

Social media and relationships definitely do not go well together. When you're going out with someone, it should be about the intimate relationship shared between the two of you – not all your followers.

If you're in the public eye there can be pressure to post about the person you're going out with. And if you haven't posted enough, people assume there's an issue and start pulling apart your relationship. That's bullshit! If you go down that route – and I have been caught like this in the past myself – you'll waste time and energy together creating some ridiculous 'couple' shots and it'll take over your life. Is that what you really want?

These days I am actively more attracted to people who barely use their social accounts and don't care about that stuff. I've definitely learned more about holding that private side of me back a bit more as I've got older.

And people who try to make their exes jealous by showing off about places they're at? Stop right now! That way madness lies.

Showing off

I did a big DJ job in Dublin recently, and when I came back and told a mate about it, their immediate reaction was, 'Why didn't you post that? It would have looked good!'

I said, 'Why would I? And who does it look good for?'

Why are we all so worried about 'looking good' and impressing people? Who really needs to see some beach pictures of me on holiday? Who needs that validation?

Women get stick for posting pics of themselves in bikinis. Men get stick for posting shots of themselves at the gym, or with their watches (that are nearly always fake) and cars. Social media can be a breeding ground for that kind of toxic masculinity.

I am certain that most of the time these pics aren't to show off to members of the opposite sex, but more about trying to prove something to their own. But it's a pressure we put ourselves under – and we shouldn't.

Trolling

I've been trolled many times over the years. And depending on the day it happens it can be laughed off or it can feel hurtful. When I first started on Capital I'd type my name in and see what was being said about me. I once read that someone hoped I'd 'die in a pool of my own AIDS'. Or I'd get upset if people were rude about my family. Now I never, ever seek out what people are saying. You realise it's all very fickle. If you're having a vulnerable day – steer clear until you're feeling more robust.

What I do like

Twitter

Mates say, 'Why do you bother? No one reads Twitter!' but I love Twitter and find some genuinely funny things on there. It's also useful for work as it lets me keep up with the news as well as telling me how people are reacting to the news. My mum never watches the news because she says it puts her in a bad place mentally.

I can see her point, but I do like to know what's going on in the world. Sometimes, though, it all gets too much. All the stuff with Boris Johnson this summer, the 'will he resign or won't he?' I just got numb to it all by the end.

Mainly, I post about silly football stuff.

The police use Twitter to help find missing people, or warn us of dangers, so we need to recognise the good aspects as well as the bad. We can't knock it all.

Highlighting awareness

There are many great aspects to social media in terms of being able to reach out to people. When I post about mental health that's 250,000 people seeing it. How else could you get a message across so quickly? And it can be inspirational when you follow people like my mate Henry Fraser, who's an amazing artist and wheelchair user who paints with his feet.

I try to follow people who make me want to better myself, not people who make me feel bad.

My nonchalant attitude toward social media goes hand in hand with me not really wanting to really be famous. It's just the job part of my life that I love, not the fame part that comes with it.

#18

DOGS

'Dogs are actually proven to make us happier'

Dogs make me happy. Fact.

There is nothing like being greeted by one as you come in the door and they're wagging their tail all pleased to see you. They give you unconditional love and no judgement and they teach you how to live in the present – you don't see a dog ever mull things over or brood obsessively, do you?

They just are. They're accepting and full of gratitude. And we could all learn a lesson from them. Mum always insists animals are here to teach us, and she could be right.

Dogs have always featured hugely in our family life.

I grew up with our pets sitting on my lap as I watched TV, sleeping at the end of my bed, and being made by Mum to take them for regular walks. I think she knew the fresh air and exercise would be good for me, and it was time to have chats.

Emma was a lovely Doberman that Mum and Dad had even before Harley and I came along. She was their baby first, and we all adored her. One of my first memories is of her large figure looming above me. Mum was always very responsible about dogs and kids – so she probably didn't leave us alone with a Doberman. You can't be too careful.

But Emma was a gentle soul, sensitive, and I'd snuggle up to her while watching TV.

THE BIG LIST OF MY LIFE

Daisy came next, she was a naughty little Shih Tzu. Very intelligent, and full of energy. I taught her to jump and play tricks. Unlike Emma, she was small enough to scoop up for cuddles and carry around.

Zac was a lovely boy, a rescue pup, and always a bit of an underdog because he was bullied by Daisy. He lived a long time, but I remember when he got poorly and Mum was in America. It was time to put him down, he was old and unwell. Mum wanted to hold on until she was back so she could say goodbye, but I was quite mature and knew it wasn't fair. Dad and I ended up taking him to be put down. Saying goodbye to much-loved pets is heartbreaking.

After I left home there was **Poppy**, a toy poodle, **Lola**, another Doberman and **Iris**, a miniature poodle who they saved from becoming dog meat from China. People who watch Celebrity Gogglebox will have seen how adorable she is.

When I lived with a girlfriend, she had a Chihuahua called **Luna** who I loved, so I know what it's like to lose 'custody' of a pet too. I can't have a dog at the minute because it wouldn't be fair with my work schedule, but I have secret fantasies about opening a dog sanctuary when I'm older.

Joe was mad about dogs, so he signed up to the BorrowMyDoggy app so he could look after other people's pets for weekends if the owners needed to go away.

At his beautiful church funeral, there was a light-hearted moment when this big Labrador barged into the middle of the ceremony and started sniffing at the coffin, bounding around happily and wagging his tail. At one point it seemed as if he was actually going to jump in the grave. It was a ridiculous, surreal scene but it made us laugh. I couldn't help but think this was some kind of comedy sign from Joe to cheer us up.

Why dogs are so good for our mental health:

- They're silly and make you laugh
- They force you to take exercise outside
- They bring a sense of community – walk a dog and you soon chat to other dog owners
- They build resilience – whatever the weather you have to pull on the right clothes and get out there
- They encourage a routine – this can really help give life a structure and a purpose
- They make you live in the present
- They give you love and affection
- Caring for something else makes you aware of how you need to take care of your own basic needs. Studies have shown that even small interactions with dogs cause the human brain to produce oxytocin, a hormone often referred to as the 'cuddle chemical'. Oxytocin increases feelings of relaxation, trust, and empathy while reducing stress and anxiety.

THE BIG LIST OF MY LIFE

LAUGHTER

'Harley is hysterical, especially when she's being silly with Mum. Those two are comedy gold'

There is nothing I enjoy more in life than having a laugh with friends. Who doesn't, right? I absolutely love making people laugh and have done ever since I was a kid doing impressions of teachers. Knowing how to 'bring the funny' is something that Joe was always talking about and trying to capture.

But there's scientific evidence that shows having a good old giggle isn't just fun – it's really good for our whole mental and physical wellbeing too. Here's eight reasons I found why we should make laughter a priority:

1. It reduces stress
Laughing lowers the levels of cortisol – the stress hormone – in our bloodstream. Less cortisol = less stress. It's also a natural pain reliever as it releases endorphins to reduce the sensation of pain.

2. Your heart will thank you
When we laugh our blood vessels dilate, helping blood to flow more easily through our veins, transporting oxygen around the body and lowering our blood pressure.

3. Aggression is reduced
Humour is often the best way to diffuse a tense situation. An off-the-cuff comment can calm things down and dampen anger and aggression, fear and rage.

4. It boosts immunity
There is really some truth in the saying 'laughter is the best medicine' as it ups your antibodies, helping fight infection and disease.

5. It makes us more sociable
Sharing funny moments – whether with colleagues, mates or even people you barely know – is a bonding experience and helps us open up to each other. According to studies, it's 30 times easier to laugh when you're in company, too.

6. Releases happy hormones
Dopamine improves our mood, adrenaline makes us more alert and receptive, and serotonin is a calming, pain-relieving endorphin. Some experts reckon chuckling helps release all three.

7. You might breathe better
There's a new yoga discipline that's been developed which focuses on laughter – apparently, big old belly tickles can help to regulate breathing and bring oxygen to the lungs.

8. It give you a six-pack
OK, OK. Maybe this is pushing it. But laughing so hard it hurts does give your abs a workout, as well as upping the production of gastric juices, which helps aid the digestive process.

THE BIG LIST OF MY LIFE

It made me think about the people who most make me laugh:

Jim Carrey

The Hollywood star was my comedy hero growing up. Watching him star in films like Ace Ventura, The Mask and Dumb and Dumber, I would just be crying with laughter watching them growing up.

I must have watched them many, many times over the years and movies like that really formed my comedy taste – basically for being incredibly silly.

Will Ferrell is another comedian I've adored since childhood. Stick on something like Anchorman or Step Brothers and it'll never fail to crack me up

Harley

She doesn't know it, because I mainly pretend she's not funny. I act like the obnoxious brother and tell her to shut up, or brush aside her gags and tell her she's embarrassing and annoying. But actually, Harley is hysterical, especially when she's being silly with Mum.

Those two are comedy gold, and sometimes I feel weirdly jealous of the fun in their relationship and the laughs they have whenever they're together.

Whereas I speak to Mum every three or four days and at length, she and Harley are on the phone a couple of times a day talking about all sorts of nonsense. They go into silly characters and have whole conversations in character and are very animated together.

Joe

The main thing I remember about Joe is laughing with him. It would always be my job to make him laugh, and I would feel it was a very good day if I'd made Joe cry with laughter. Often it was something random that would most tickle him.

We'd go to maybe the last viewing of a cinema, at one o'clock in the morning in Leicester Square and there'd be hardly anyone there.

One evening we went to some terrible Jason Statham movie (no disrespect to Jason, but it was bad). We were the only two people there – apart from Brian May from Queen sat in front of us with his former EastEnders actress wife Anita Dobson.

Joe found this hilarious, especially when Brian turned around, nodded at us and then put up his rockstar fingers – no joke – he gave us the bulls horns. So Joe starts giggling uncontrollably, and we're sitting there staring at the back of Brian May's gigantic hair.

It felt absurd. Then the film started and Brian May turned round and shushes us really loudly. Well, that just set Joe off even more.

Next thing I know he's whipped out his camera – flash! – and he's actually taken a picture of Brian May telling us off. 'What are you doing?' demands Brian, which was fair enough. But it caused more giggles.

We ended up sloping out before the end.

THE BIG LIST OF MY LIFE

RELIGION

This is another one I've put on my list...

It's generally thought that religious people have higher levels of happiness than non-religious people. I can well imagine that having a strong belief and faith in God, as well as feeling part of a real community, might help many people.

I don't have a faith of my own, though, and I grew up in a non-religious family. Being raised in north London, I had more Jewish friends than Christian or Muslim ones, but Mum and Dad always instilled in us to be accepting of everyone's faith and beliefs.

They always thought it was important to understand different religions and encouraged us to make friends with different people. I know that if I had ever turned around to them and said I wanted to explore any faith they would have been totally up for that.

As it happened, I was quite anti-religion as a teenager. When we were told to say prayers at school, which was Church of England, I was the person in class who said, 'I don't believe in God, so I'm not going to say that.' We'd get told to go to chapel and I'd say I didn't want to.

So it might surprise you to learn that I actually got an A* for my Religious Studies GCSE. It was one of the few subjects I genuinely loved, and mainly thanks to the fact I had an amazing teacher. Mr Wiles was a tall, imposing man with a big beard and huge hands who taught religious studies and was head of my house. He had a knack of making everyone feel like they had a voice, and he treated all the kids with respect.

I loved the fact in his classes we were allowed to argue a point, and never felt like there was a 'wrong answer'. His classes were thought-provoking and helped all of us to find a voice.

But the one thing that really changed my mind about religion was when I was 19 and I lost my friend Patrick. He was part of our friendship group at prep school and then at secondary school too.

The only person I'd lost by that stage of my life were my grandparents, but they were old. Patrick was the first person my age I knew who had died.

He was killed in a car crash. As a teenager it was hard to make sense of a tragedy like that. He was from a big eastern European family, with lots of siblings, and they were all very Catholic.

His funeral was a very religious ceremony. At the end I went up to Patrick's dad, Jack, in tears and told him how sorry I was for his loss. I remember Jack just looking back at me, smiling and saying, 'That's God's plan.' It clearly wasn't what any of that family wanted, but it was like they'd accepted it was meant to happen.

Part of me thought this acceptance was a bit crazy – he'd just lost his son! But the other part of me thought, this is amazing, to have such a strong faith that it can make you take this horrific thing and see it and understand it from a different viewpoint.

It was that moment when I came to really respect religion, and I changed my whole vibe on it.

For most of my life, Mum was always interested in spirituality rather than a firm religion.

THE BIG LIST OF MY LIFE

I remember as a kid having a shaman come to the house in the middle of the night, or someone to do Reiki or bring a crystal ball. She loves all those New Age therapies, and while she avoided Tarot card readings as she never wanted to hear anything negative, she loved Angel card readings, which are supposed to be more motivational and inspirational.

Recently, my mum got baptised, which meant a lot to her. Despite not being religious earlier in life she is finding it more of a comfort now, and I support her wholeheartedly.

I'm pretty open about exploring all that. But I can't see myself ever committing to any one faith.

#21 FOOTBALL

'Being able to watch a game is the best form of escapism for me. For those 90 minutes, I genuinely do not care about anything else'

Football means the world to me. If I'm not watching it or playing it I'll be following it or thinking about it. It's a bit of an obsession.

I love everything about it: the teamwork, dedication, discipline, resilience and the excitement. I've had some of the best moments of my life watching games, and being on the pitch with my mates is the one place I can really be myself.

It's the one activity and passion that really keeps my sanity.

Watching footy (victory to Dad – a Gooner for life)

My dad and his dad were lifelong Arsenal supporters, and coming from north London, I guess it was always my destiny to support them. And Dad made sure of that.

He took me to the old stadium at Highbury for the first time when I was four to see Arsenal v Coventry.

'You'll never forget this first time,' he said, walking me up the steps. And he was right. I can still remember marvelling at how green the pitch was, like someone had taken a highlighter pen and drawn it, it didn't look real.

THE BIG LIST OF MY LIFE

That vibe you get at a game is unique, the energy from the crowds makes you buzz like nothing else I've experienced. The way everyone there is sharing the same emotions, that sweet anticipation before the match begins, you're all in it together and it's so powerful. You're part of a club, you're part of the family, but it feels bigger than that too.

After going to watch that match, Dad started taking me to Alexandra Palace to learn how to play, and we'd have a five-a-side 'World Cup' tournament each week. All the kids wanted to be England, but weirdly I was obsessed with being France and Holland. Funnily enough, later in life when I played for Soccer Aid, I was always happy to be in the Rest of the World team. I'm very patriotic but, when it comes to football, it's a bigger love than that. I want to know more about all the best players from all over the world.

The very first game I remember watching on telly and being properly invested in was England versus Colombia in the 1998 World Cup. I was five and can still feel the excitement of watching David Beckham score.

Afterwards, Beckham did this celebration move where he thrusted his hips – basically it looked like he was shagging the air. I had no idea what shagging was back then, but I thought it was a very cool move, so I started doing the same every time I scored at Ally Pally. God knows what the other parents made of that. Then I remember watching England versus Argentina in that same tournament, seeing David Beckham being given the red card, and feeling the utter disappointment of losing.

Before I was a truly committed Gooner, though, there was a stage where my parents' friends were trying to get me to support different teams. After that World Cup, my dad's friend, Willie, got me a signed David Beckham shirt. I was over the moon.

But Dad was dying inside seeing me running around in this Manchester United top.

Then Yog came over and asked me who my favourite player was. 'Michael Owen,' I proudly declared. So then Yog (who supported Arsenal too, but not passionately) gave me a Michael Owen Liverpool shirt.

Dad was far from thrilled about that either. So in the year when Arsenal won the Double – both the FA Cup and the Premier League – Dad decided to make sure I knew who my team really was.

He took me, Harley and Mum to the after-match celebrations, wearing all the kit, with the car fully decked out with red flags and a huge inflatable trophy. Dad put me on top of his shoulders to watch the team drive around on an open-top bus at Highbury corner, and he pointed them out and firmly told me, 'That's your team, Ro.' And that was it. Arsenal have been my team ever since. Victory to Dad.

Football became such a great bond for me and Dad as well as Grandad, his dad. Up until Grandad's death in 2009 he would call me on the landline as soon as the whistle had blown after every single Arsenal match and ask me all about tactics and what I thought, like I was in some manager's interview. I loved it.

Being able to watch a game is the best form of escapism for me. For those 90 minutes, I genuinely do not care about anything else.

And nothing beats that collective feeling, when you're able to share in emotions – as a kid I sat with grown men in tears at matches and I've now become that grown man in tears sometimes. It's such a great release.

People who aren't into the game might not get it, but I

honestly think there are skills you learn about all of life from being a football supporter.

It's helped me as a person understand things like loss, and it's helped me understand things that sometimes the world doesn't go the way you want it to. It teaches you resilience. If you lose you lose, you just pick yourself back up.

One of my best ever memories is of taking my dad for his 60th to the final of the Euros last year. I was offered a ticket for live sponsorship but I said no, I didn't want to be in some corporate box. So I paid silly amounts to take my dad and be in the stands. I knew there would be no better present in the world than having that shared memory. We had England shirts and bucket hats on and it was bloody amazing. When England scored that first goal, Dad got so involved I looked up and saw him rolling down the stairs in the stands with other fans in pure elation! At the end of the match when we lost, we had a little cry and hug.

For a long time Dad and I had Arsenal season tickets but we stopped when the team stopped spending money on players. We felt like why should we spend the money if they're not? A very passive aggressive decision, I admit.

People who only watch football during the big England games say things like, 'I don't know how you deal with losing, it's horrible, how do you stand it?' But real fans know full well you take the highs and lows in your stride.

And it teaches us the importance of loyalty, too.

I remember Mum saw I was very downcast after Arsenal lost one time. 'Why don't you just support another team then, like Chelsea?' she cheerfully suggested.

I was horrified. Your team is your team, they're like your family, you don't desert them.

What I also love about football is that it's an international language, I can meet people from all around the world, and if they say they're an Arsenal fan, then we're suddenly chatting away.

If you don't know what to say to a bloke you don't know or if there's an awkward silence, you ask if they've seen a match and – boom! – you're off.

Men aren't always the best talkers, and what I really want to do is get more men talking. And if football is a way of opening up for them, then it's an easy win.

Football does my mental health so much good. Being part of a tribe. I feel I belong.

Playing footy (Netflix and Skill...)

As a kid, of course, I fantasised about being a professional footballer. Despite the fact I've only ever rated myself as a six-and-a-half or seven out of 10 on the pitch.

I wasn't bad when I was seven or eight, but when I hit 13 I saw how good the other boys were getting and realised I was never going to be a pro. I was slowing down. My legs grew long quickly, and they started aching more, and I got a bit of puppy fat hitting puberty. It's all about how your body grows at that stage and mine wasn't turning into an elite athlete's, alas!

But it wasn't what I'd describe as a devastating realisation knowing the pro dream was over, for me I just loved playing and being part of this family and community you feel joined to when you walk into the dressing rooms each week. I just loved having that human connection through a game.

Most of the time I'd moan like hell about having to wear my school blazer, but as soon as we went to an away game at another school, I loved pulling it on and wearing it with pride to show where I belonged.

I've been playing with my mates from school in a team we rather cheesily call 'Netflix and Skill' for the past four years and it's genuinely my saviour.

There's nine of us in the WhatsApp group, and Wednesday nights are sacred to me.

I've turned down dates and I've turned down good money for jobs before, all because I don't want to miss my weekly kickabout. I love them and I live for them.

####

'After the game I got him to open up, and it all came out. He was worried about work, he'd split from his girlfriend… and had even had thoughts about taking his own life'

####

Netflix and Skill started out because of Patrick, the school friend we had who died in a car crash. His dad suggested we play a game in honour of him against the football team Patrick used to play for.

Bearing in mind their team played together every week, and us lot hadn't played since school, we fully expected to get a drubbing. But we all just knew each other. I hadn't seen some of the lads for years, they'd gone off to university and things, but as soon as we were on the pitch it was like we remembered exactly what it was like to play with each other. We could anticipate everyone's moves and every shot and position. We had this connection which was weird but wonderful. Against the odds we ended up totally battering the other side and having a complete blast. So we decided to do it every week.

It's not just a chance to exercise together and let off steam, it's an important chance to really connect. Recently, I noticed something was up with a good friend. I've known him since he was eight. He just seemed lost on the pitch. I was watching him running and he was getting lost, almost not realising where he was. I knew something wasn't right.

'What's going on? You're not here,' I grilled.

'What are you talking about?' he snapped.

But then after the game I pursued it, I got him to open up, and it all came out. He was worried about work, he'd split from his girlfriend, he just wasn't in a good place and had even had thoughts about taking his own life.

As shocked and upset as I felt that things had gotten so bad for him, I was so glad I was able to talk to him, and that he had opened up. But that's the power of playing together regularly. You can check in on your mates. Football can be that outlet for people, for sure. When you're being super, super physical your emotions can run high and sometimes, you might feel like you can speak honestly. It really does help to talk.

For me personally, playing football helps me feel like a normal person, it puts me on a level playing field. I'm not Roman Kemp, I'm just a guy having a kickabout with his mates.

There have been so many times where I've noticed that the other team will try to go for me, because of who I am, or who they want to go back and tell their mates they had a go at me. In regular life, if I'm in a bar or something, if someone's shouting my name or calling me a prick, I'm not able to say anything. I have to shut up.

But on a football pitch, I can safely and acceptably stand up for myself. The only time in life when I ever feel aggression is when I'm on the football pitch, and it's a great outlet for me. It's like that for a lot of guys.

When I'm playing football, I'm totally absorbed, I feel like I can really be myself. I want other guys to have that feeling of being themselves – whether it's on the football pitch, or at the gym or any other place you feel at home, being able to have that release is so powerful.

My mate Charlie often tells me he has no confidence, yet as I always say to him, when he goes on a football pitch he walks on and he's a leader, winning every call. I'm trying to get him to channel that a bit more in his life.

After the game, all of us always go to the pub. And if someone says they're not coming, we always ask 'Why?' Often it means something is up.

I've never drank alcohol at any of those times in the pub because I'm working the next morning. The pub part is important, but it's not about boozing for me. I stick to a Diet Coke or soda and blackcurrant. It's all about being together and being sociable with my mates.

And it means everything to me.

My dream team

For years I longed to work on Sky's Soccer AM. They'd never let me of course – but getting to appear on the show with Dad was a real dream come true.

While I've accepted I'll never earn my living playing the game, I still find it hard to accept I'll never be a sports presenter! Well, maybe one day, I can dream…

Anyway, as it's my book, I'd like to indulge myself (if it makes me feel better then why not?) with my all-time fantasy team line-up.

Here's who I'd pick:

1. Goalie – David Seaman
What a career! Who else could pull off that hair and moustache? As a kid he came into our school, York House, doing some promotion. The teacher asked if anyone had any questions, and my hand was the first up. He'd just made one of the best saves of his life and I asked, 'Do you think it was over the line?' David laughed. I kept asking more questions, everyone else was too scared but I was in my element. I ended up meeting David a few times, when I heard him call me 'little Roman' I was beyond made up that he knew my name.

2. Defence – Kolo Toure
To try to get me reading as a kid, Dad started giving me the sports section of the newspapers as he knew I'd be interested. One day, when I was 13, I came out of school and Dad was there to pick me up. He handed me the newspaper that day and said, 'Check out what Arsenal are up to.' They were playing against Villareal in the Champions League semi-final, so I kept flipping through to find the page, and when I did Dad had paperclipped two tickets to the game that night. I can remember exactly where I was on the school driveway as I found them. Toure scored in that game and we won, so I will always remember him.

3. Defence – Roberto Carlos
Brazil is the greatest footballing nation ever, and I remember seeing him play in 1998 and doing the most meticulous bending

free-kick I've ever seen. It literally defied the laws of physics and I was blown away. I spent the rest of my childhood, in fact my life, trying to recreate that free-kick.

4. Defence – Sol Campbell
Sol got so much stick from Tottenham fans when he transferred from them over to Arsenal. I'd never seen someone get so much hate like that. That was the first time I learned what the word 'Judas' meant. It was 2006 and we made it to the Champions League final and he scored and we went a goal up. In the end we lost 2-1. But for those 78 minutes it was glorious. I've never celebrated a goal so much in my life.

5. Midfield – David Beckham
How could I not include Beckham? I grew up in the generation where we watched him become a superstar in front of our eyes. He was The Man. When he had his blond mohawk with frosted tips I got Mum to do it to me. (I also sported a mullet for a while like Fernando Torres, which my mates still rinse me about.)

I remember the first time I went to the David Beckham Academy with Charlie, it was a London soccer camp in the summer and the man himself was there. It was a big, big moment for me, aged 11. I was the kid that couldn't stop talking to him. He'd just moved to Real Madrid so I was asking him all about that. He looked the same as he did on telly, he sounded the same, and here he was surrounded by all these kids and he was just a lovely, normal guy.

Many years later, I had to interview David's son Cruz on Capital once via Zoom and David popped up in the background and said, 'Hello Roman.'

It was very cool and surreal.

6. Midfield – Patrick Vieira

An incredible midfielder, Patrick was also captain when I was growing up. Arsene Wenger brought him over in 1996, and I was so impressed by this skinny, elegant guy who stood at an imposing 6ft 4ins tall. He was a hot-headed, aggressive mean machine, and one of the most red-carded players, but it was a pure thrill watching him in action.

7. Midfield – Zinedine Zidane

One of the greatest players of all time in my book. The skills he invented became the ones I then had to try and learn myself at school.

He had the grace of a dancer doing a 360 around the ball. Unbelievable. He was one of the famous Galacticos I became obsessed with.

I remember watching him in the Italy versus France 2006 World Cup final with my grandparents and Dad. It turned out to be the last game Zidane ever played – and he was sent off in extra time for headbutting the chest of Italian defender Marco Materazzi. My nan was so animated – she was desperate to see it kick off between them!

I couldn't believe he was throwing away his biggest moment being sent off in a World Cup final. Dad had always drummed it into me not to react on the pitch.

I remember, aged 14, getting punched in the face as a kid when I was going for a header. I saw the kid who did it and later, when he barely had the ball, I went through him. Right in front of my dad. This kid was hurt on the floor and Dad had me subbed off, then had a massive go at me as to why I couldn't do that.

Sometimes that passion just gets the better of you.

8. Midfield – Marc Overmars

Overmars was a Dutch player and the first person I ever had on the back of my shirt when I was nine. I don't know why I wanted him so badly on my shirt really, a foreign player not an English one, but he was amazing.

He was a stylish, dangerous player. My shirt was a horrible yellow one, because Arsenal were being sponsored by JCB at the time. I barely took it off so it probably stank half the time. I got nicknamed 'Overmars' because it was what I always wore when I played at Ally Pally.

9. Forward – Michael Owen

At that first World Cup I really remember, back in 1998, the standout player was an 18-year-old Michael Owen, and he became the person I wanted to be. I was so fascinated by this gifted young kid I didn't even care that England went out, I just thought he was fantastic. And his youth made it all the more impressive.

10. Forward – Thierry Henry

In my opinion, Henry's the best striker we've ever had in the history of the Premier League.

I remember the day he joined and for so long, week in, week out, my happiness – along with so many other Arsenal fans – would rely on him scoring. Literally, that man brought me so much joy and happiness.

My dad always says he had Ian Wright and Charlie George to hero worship, but for me it was Thierry Henry. And now his statue stands at the new stadium.

I met him once when he was involved in the Prince's Trust, and OMG, I've never been more nervous in my life. Ever. I was

25 and had proper sweaty palms and a rash going up my neck as I stood in front of this incredibly suave Frenchman. I was starstruck in a way I've never before been. Utter legend.

11. Forward – Ronaldo Luís Nazário de Lima

The original Ronaldo was the best in the world for me. I've always been fascinated by Brazil, and this guy came from nothing to being the most gifted player on the planet. He was just untouchable. Pure sunshine to watch.

For Dad it was Maradona, for me it will always be Ronaldo.

Dad surprised me when I was five or six with these R9 Nike football boots, they were blue and yellow and my most treasured item of clothing.

THE BIG LIST OF MY LIFE

THE ROYAL FAMILY

'Prince Harry tried to coax me into firing a water balloon at Prince William. 'What is going on?' I laughed. Prince Harry said 'Aim a bit to the left.' Who am I aiming for?' I asked, and he said 'My brother!"

I love the Royal Family and I can get weirdly very patriotic at times. Perhaps that surprises you, but I think we all realised after what's happened this year just how important the monarchy is to our identity in Britain. The Queen will remain a legend forever in my eyes. Talk about a strong woman. But when it comes to mental health, I especially respect the fact that Prince William and Prince Harry have been so open in the past about their own struggles at times. It's brave and was an important progression in getting the conversations going.

One of the strongest memories that I have as a kid was being sat down and watching my mum in tears watching Princess Diana's funeral. Yog was a firm friend of Diana so there was a close connection there. And how could anyone not be desperately moved by seeing these young boys mourn for their beloved mum?

I've been lucky enough to meet and work with several members of the Royal Family over the years.

ROMAN KEMP – ARE YOU REALLY OK?

The first person I met was Prince William in 2015. I think the Duke of Cambridge is amazing for the way he's talked about his own mental health over the years, to have someone of that status being frank about their struggles was brave and deserves massive respect.

We were teamed up with Rio Ferdinand and some others back then for work on a programme called Heads Together, and I took my mate Charlie along too. Charlie had lost his mum to breast cancer when he was young, and I had this surreal, very moving moment of watching my best mate talk to Prince William. Both had gone through that terrible loss and grief so young and had it shape their lives. The Royals endure all the same human hardships the rest of us do, but have to cope with them so publicly. I don't envy them at all.

We chatted about mental health, and I think they are really genned up on that as a family. They're good people.

They might have to live by strict codes, but I've always found them off duty to be extremely normal and down to earth and relaxed company.

Before I met Prince William for the first time for that mental health charity, I was given a whole protocol to follow. It was a regal situation, and I started worrying whether I was meant to bow and what I was supposed to do. I was told to address him as Your Highness and advised where to stand, how to act, all that sort of thing.

But there was a football match on telly going on in the corner of the room and it had just finished. It was a bit of a crazy game and Prince William came walking over to say hello just as it was wrapping up. Everything I'd been advised on Royal protocol suddenly went out the window and so the first words I said to our future king were, 'Fucking hell mate, that was mad!'

I then panicked, worrying I'd just sworn at him! Luckily, he just laughed. After that, formalities were forgotten, it would have been weird to go back and stop calling him mate.

The next year I got a letter from Prince Harry inviting me to work at the Palace as a DJ for one of the garden parties which was open to some of the public.

I took my mum as I knew she would be so excited. She honestly couldn't believe it when I announced, 'We're gonna go for a party in the park at Buckingham Palace!'

We still have a picture of us both beaming.

I think it was one of my mum's proudest days. She got all dressed up and looked beautiful. For me, that's a moment that I'll never forget. I've got a lot of unforgettable moments with my dad, through working together, but it was lovely to have that one special moment with Mum.

One of the most surprising things was that it wasn't remotely glamorous inside the Palace. We were given a bedroom upstairs to get ready in, and as soon as we walked in all I could think was, 'This is just like my nan's house!'

It had a single bed pushed up against the corner of this tiny little room, and terrible old-lady style wallpaper.

In the corner of the room was a rather sad-looking trouser press. There was Jo Malone hand wash, but it sat on a basic sink that was just attached to the wall, and then a really old-school TV was sat in the corner of the room.

We thought it was quite funny and not what we expected. But also just very normal. Which the family is at heart.

I was playing some rap, a Migos track, and Prince Harry strolled over.

'Oh, I really liked this song,' he said.

Then he grins at me.

'Er, just double checking, you've got the radio edit, right? I didn't want the ACTUAL lyrics ('Fore she fuck me/give me top, top') going out at the Queen's house...'

Luckily, I did have the clean version.

It felt surreal to be there. I'd gone from creating YouTube videos in my bedroom the year before to DJ-ing to the crowds at Buckingham Palace.

Later, Prince Harry beckoned me over. 'Roman, come here,' he said. Kate Middleton was there and there was a slingshot in the middle of them. They had a bucket filled with water balloons, and were pinging them into the crowd from a balcony. Prince Harry tried to coax me into firing a water balloon at Prince William.

'What is going on?' I laughed.

Prince Harry said, 'Aim a bit to the left.'

Who am I aiming for?' I asked, and he said, 'My brother!'

I didn't want to be done for treason, I joked – but Prince Harry has a cheeky sense of humour you can't help warming to.

When Prince Harry first announced he was off to America, I thought it was a shame for Britain, but from a personal level I was quite pleased for him.

It was a move he clearly felt was something he wanted to do, and though it was a massive deal for the Royal Family, you can only have respect for someone for doing what they believe is right in that moment.

Him and Prince William went through such a huge trauma as kids, and the fact they've acknowledged that openly sends a very powerful message to all of us to talk more about these things and to seek help when you need it. It's not a sign of weakness.

I am grateful to both of them for that.

THE BIG LIST OF MY LIFE

The Platinum Jubilee gig

Of course I was thrilled to get asked to present some of the BBC coverage for the Platinum Jubilee celebrations this June. And now, looking back, I feel even more privileged to have been part of those historic celebrations. But man, did that give me a strong sense of imposter syndrome! Millions of people would be watching. Was I really up to it?

It's jobs like that that get me thinking, 'Am I doing this because they think I'm good enough? Or am I being offered this because they just think I'm hot right now?' I can't help doubting myself sometimes. But I had to try and put those doubts to one side and accept it, and make the most of it. It was an honour to take part, and I loved it.

At the afterparty at Bucks Palace I managed to make another classic Kemp blunder in front of the Duchess of Cambridge.

The party was held in the 'throne room' no less, and it was all very upper-class when I literally just bumped into Kate and got a bit nervous, and then I blurted out that I felt a bit silly all dressed up. She kindly told me I looked nice and smart, and that I'd done a fantastic job that day.

I'd had a couple of drinks by then and I got all flustered and said to the Duchess of Cambridge, 'Yeah, you look well fit too.'

I was mortified that I'd just told the future Queen of England that she was 'fit'. Luckily, she laughed.

In my defence, I think you're granted a pass to get a bit nervous and say the wrong thing in these circumstances with these people.

Kate sometimes comes under fire for coming across as 'aloof'. But that isn't how she is at all. She's simply very nice, very friendly, and very down to earth.

The Queen

I really feel like that the Platinum Jubilee celebrations weren't just 70 years of celebrating the Queen's incredible achievements, it was as much about the public thanking her for all she did. She essentially lived her entire life for her country. People are quick to say, she had everything, she had a nice life. But it's not normal, is it? Having all that duty piled on your shoulders. She didn't ask for it, she just had to graciously get on with it.

She coped with her own battles and she led the country for 70 years doing good things for people. Half the good work the Royals do we never know about, it's quietly carried out behind the scenes.

So I'm very proud of the Queen and what she represented, like I'm very proud of my country.

Of course there are some family 'dysfunctions' within the Royal lot. But show me a family that doesn't have those! The Queen always protected her family, just like I would in that position.

THE BIG LIST OF MY LIFE

#23

TELLY

> *'I loved the show Gogglebox instantly, but Dad was hesitant about going on it. 'Nah, I don't think so Ro, I don't want people in the house, seeing me scratching my bits and all that"*

I actually always fancied being behind the camera a bit more than being in front of it, which must seem a strange comment for someone whose gurning mug is on the telly quite a lot, I know. When I'm relaxing at home the only thing I really watch is documentaries. I love learning new things, but I don't read that much, so watching stuff on TV is how I educate myself.

First taste of TV

It was Dad who got me onto the small screen for the first time.

'Right Ro, we're making a TV show together, and it involves flying a plane,' he cheerily announced one morning in our kitchen. 'Let's do it!'

I was a slightly surly 14-year-old. 'Absolutely not,' I replied, munching on my toast.

'Too late, I've already signed us up,' he laughed. Dad is a mild-mannered man, but when he wants to do something he can be quite determined.

It was a Channel 5 TV show called Dangerous Adventures

for Boys, and in our episode Dad and I had to take to the air to find out what it was like to be a pilot in the Battle of Britain.

It's never about the cash for Dad, or for ratings, or for raising his profile, he basically just fancied having a go at flying, and it was a father-and-son adventure so I needed to be on board too. To be fair, he probably knew it would be a chance for us to have some bonding time as well.

But for me, at 14, when I was at my peak of trying to be cool at school, it all sounded mortifying. Being on telly in some cringe show with your own dad just wasn't cool. Especially as I had a fear of flying back then. The idea of getting into the cockpit of a WW2 aeroplane was my worst nightmare.

I turned up reluctantly on the first day of filming, a bit like Kevin the Teenager. I looked just like a cross between Kelly Osbourne and Ellen DeGeneres at the time. My hair was dyed blondish and plastered around my slightly chubby face. I thought I looked the business but it's fairly shocking to look back on now!

But slowly, I got into making the episode. We were taught how to dogfight in WW2 – and I loved it. It was an amazing feeling, being hundreds of feet in the air, doing manoeuvres and waving to my dad across the sky.

It was also my first opportunity to be on camera, and my first chance to get to interview someone on film as we had to speak to veteran pilots and hear their tales.

Amazingly, Dad kind of just let me do it. He handed over the microphone and the responsibility. I think we were both surprised how naturally I took to it. It felt easy, not awkward.

Watching Dad taught me a lot on that show. Watching how he handled things – from walking into a room to meet all the camera crew; making sure you say hello to everyone; looking everyone in the eye; always remembering to say thank you – all those important things, Dad knew they mattered.

'You've seen me do it, now you show me,' he said, handing over the microphone. And that was the first time that I realised, 'Okay, I'm carrying the Kemp name, and I need to walk on set and act like a professional, like my dad.'

I don't feel under pressure to emulate Dad's success. But the one thing I feel I have to do is be a decent person, like he is. That's the most important thing, and I think that's the key to longevity in any career.

The best thing about making that show was that I'll always have a memory that I can share with Dad forever.

Million Pound Drop

The next time we were on TV together didn't go so well. I was in my late teens when we went on Davina McCall's game show, and were trying to win for charity.

We put a bunch of money on knowing a certain answer.

I was completely cocky and made that classic error of failing to read the question properly. So when the question came up 'Which one of these isn't an Olympic sport?' I misread it as which one was an Olympic sport, and straight away went for 'Skeleton'. We put a million quid on it, it was the first question, and I totally bollocksed it up.

I felt a total dick going back into school after that.

Celebrity Gogglebox

Dad and I have worked together many times since then. I love working with Dad, there's just a natural ease between us.

I loved the show Gogglebox instantly, but Dad was hesitant about going on it. 'Nah, I don't think so Ro, I don't want people in the house, seeing me scratching my bits and all that.' But I managed to persuade him, just as he'd persuaded me as a teen.

I knew it would be fun, and I wanted everyone to see how hysterical Dad is too.

That banter is exactly what we're like in real life.

At first he didn't feel comfortable, he was used to following a script or wheeling out an anecdote for a chat show, but he didn't like the idea of just being himself. He worried what people would think of him.

But he soon got the hang of it and now I can't stop him talking about inappropriate things.

One time he made a comment to me and said, 'You know what I would do if left alone in that house?'

I looked at him blank. He chirps, 'Wank'.

I couldn't quite believe he'd said that, but I guess I wanted him to come out of his shell…

Martin & Roman's Weekend Best

Hosting the magazine show together is a nice job.

But it was interesting because for the first time the roles had changed. Dad wasn't the presenter and I had to coach him how to do things such as ad-lib and be a bit less robotic. That took a little bit of getting used to! He said he knew his place when he saw that I'd been given dressing room one and he'd been relegated to dressing room two.

Because of the dyslexia he was left with after the brain tumour, sometimes he struggled with the autocue.

'Oh you've got more lines than me,' he'll say, acting hurt.

'That's because you keep fucking it up Dad!' I'll laugh. 'And we want to get the job done and go home.'

For some reason I'm quite good at reading the autocue, but everyone thinks it is because if you ask me two minutes later what I've said, I've no idea. It's in one ear and out the other with me.

The One Show

It's a lovely job being on The One Show.

But I took an absolute hammering on Twitter earlier this year for one of my appearances outside Buckingham Palace in the build-up to the Jubilee celebrations.

I'd misread an email, and thought I was heading to the TV studio for hair and make-up. I imagined I was just gonna do a small segment – you know, 'we're doing this, and the ballot's going to be open and you can get your tickets' and all those types of things. I was in my tracksuit as I was off to play football later. I got in the taxi they sent me, but then it started taking a few turns I didn't recognise.

Suddenly, it dawned on me that we were arriving at Buckingham Palace, not the studio, and there were several armed guards asking for ID. I had no make-up, my hair was all skew-whiff and I looked like Boris Johnson.

Someone rummaged up an old suit from the Palace's lost property, but I looked a right state, and I got slagged off on Twitter for not wearing a tie and having hair that looked like my nana had styled it with a food blender!

Not my finest moment, I admit – but luckily they've kept me on the show.

Other TV programmes I've popped up on are...

ROMAN KEMP – ARE YOU REALLY OK?

Xtra Factor

While I was busying working through the ranks at Capital, a nice lady at ITV called Shu Green was trying to help me get a foot in the door on TV. She really believed in me for some reason, and kept encouraging me. And I got to host a little segment on the Xtra Factor, with Rylan and Matt Edmondson.

It was a great chance to get experience of live TV, and I learned a lot from Rylan about how to hold myself. He's really funny but also very nice to everyone on set.

Take Me Out

Paddy McGuinness brought me out after the very handsome rugby player Tom Evans had been on. So nearly all the girls turned their lights off for me!

Oh well, I got to roll out some of my impressions – Kermit the Frog, David Attenborough and Arnold Schwarzenegger all got an outing, I seem to remember.

I'm A Celebrity

Although it caused me a fair amount of stress beforehand, the whole should/shouldn't I do it, going into the jungle was one of the best things I've ever done. I had the happiest time of my life in there.

I'd been first asked to do the show three years earlier. I said no back then because it just didn't feel it was the right time. I would have been there as Martin Kemp's son. It felt I hadn't done enough to deserve to be Roman.

In my own right.

But by 2019 I'd been working at Capital for three years. I told myself that even if the rest of the UK didn't get it, I knew I'd have some listeners backing me.

Life just felt beautifully simple in the jungle.

I was going in with some huge names – Caitlyn Jenner was one of the big celebrities on the planet, and I'd grown up worshipping Ian Wright, so it was like having a hero there, and James Haskell was this beast of a man and a real gentle giant. But if anything I was more starstruck by the set than the people as I was such a longtime fan of the show.

I always loved I'm A Celebrity, since the very first series Tony Blackburn won. It always started on a Sunday night, and I'd have to get in the bath and get everything sorted out for school before I was allowed to watch it.

Like Mum, I'm a born worrier. So I scrutinised all my social media beforehand, paranoid something would be taken out of context and deemed offensive and I'd be trolled. I wanted to do my parents proud and not bring shame to the Kemp name. I had a girlfriend at the time and I didn't want to let her down either.

I put so much pressure on myself worrying about going on the show.

I chatted to Dad, he just said to me: 'Look, Ro, just go in, enjoy it. Don't get divided up into splinter groups, and just stay on the fence about everything. Keep out of arguments, it's none of your business.'

I tried to follow his advice, but on the second episode, I managed to upset the Radio One DJ Adele Roberts.

We'd lost everyone's personal items in a challenge. Jacqueline Jossa had lost photos of her kids, Ian Wright had lost music that reminded him of his family. One of the few people who hadn't lost theirs was Adele. And when I asked her what her personal item was, she said it was a picture of Jane McDonald, the slightly cheesy singer. I couldn't help but laugh that we'd managed to save that. But Adele was upset and called me 'prejudiced'.

Well, she's a lovely lady and I felt mortified I'd upset her. But I was also bloody terrified that spelt the end of my career. As a white, straight guy I was suddenly terrified of being called 'prejudiced' on national TV by a black, gay woman.

####

> *'I just didn't want my life back. I didn't want to be Roman Kemp who struggles with trying to keep his mental health in check. In the jungle I was just Ro and I was really happy'*

####

Harley said that every night she watched me on the show she felt physically sick in case I did something stupid.

I imagined my whole career crashing and burning.

I've always been an emotional person, and I worked myself into a state worrying I'd upset or embarrassed Adele.

I will always be the first person to apologise if I've upset someone. I immediately said sorry and that I hadn't intended any malice, but she was having none of it.

The next day, after that episode had been aired, I was then voted to do a trial – against Adele. So I panicked and everyone thought I was some racist, homophobe.

But it turned out to be fine. The real reason why I was voted for the trial was more likely due to the fact my dad had tweeted saying, 'I really want to see my boy eat kangaroo dick.' Once I'd got over the Adele fallout, I relaxed and forgot about everything outside.

I made some great friends there.

Kate Garraway was a bit like a mum in there towards me, she's very level-headed and kind.

I spent hours talking to Caitlyn Jenner. She's one of the most inspirational people I've ever met. Formerly known as Bruce Jenner, the Olympic gold medal-winning decathlete was offered the role of Superman, but turned it down because she knew at the time she wanted to transition. That is brave.

I really clicked with James Haskell, too. I loved our deep, open chats about life. He's very empathetic, he loves understanding people and always gave others the floor to be able to express themselves, which I really respected. I was upset he was cast in an unflattering, oafish light on the show because that wasn't how he was at all. When he got eliminated I actually cried, which I now see is ridiculous. But all your emotions are heightened there.

I love Ian Wright, but I found him difficult. He has an amazing outlook on life, but there were some days when he made me feel like I was the person who should have left. Ian can be like two different people, he can wake up one morning and be the happiest guy in the world, or he can wake up and just won't talk to anyone. But I tried not to overthink that.

I never expected to win, but I was completely made up and delighted to have had all these amazing experiences and make it to the final three!

I remember walking across that bridge, and doing my interview straightaway, where they show you your best bits. I felt completely overwhelmed by the cameras and lights and people everywhere. I felt dazed, like I couldn't recognize anyone that was there, even my girlfriend I didn't really speak to.

It was a harsh welcome back to reality.

And while Ant and Dec were busy interviewing Jacqueline Jossa, who came first, and Corrie star Andy 'Kirky' Whyment, I was honest to God curled up in a ball crying! I was so scared of coming out.

People were calling me Ro, and all of a sudden I felt like I wasn't defined by my surname, I was just 'Ro' – which is what all my mates call me.

It was like this weird, existential moment and I had to be pulled into a room where a therapist talked to me.

I think it was just this relief I felt. I felt accepted.

When I got back home my mates had organised a surprise party for 100 people at Mahiki, a bar in central London. Joe was there, everyone was there. I got wind of it and really didn't want to go. Charlie and Matt picked me up and I cried in the car. They talked me down and I went for a drink and it was fine, but I couldn't deal with everyone looking at me.

I just didn't want my life back. I didn't want to be Roman Kemp who struggles with trying to get his mental health in check. In the jungle I was just Ro and I was really happy.

It was autumn 2015 when I first met Joe at Capital. With him by my side, I learned quickly, he was an excellent teacher. Even now it's Joe's voice I hear in my head, telling me what I've done wrong, how I could be better

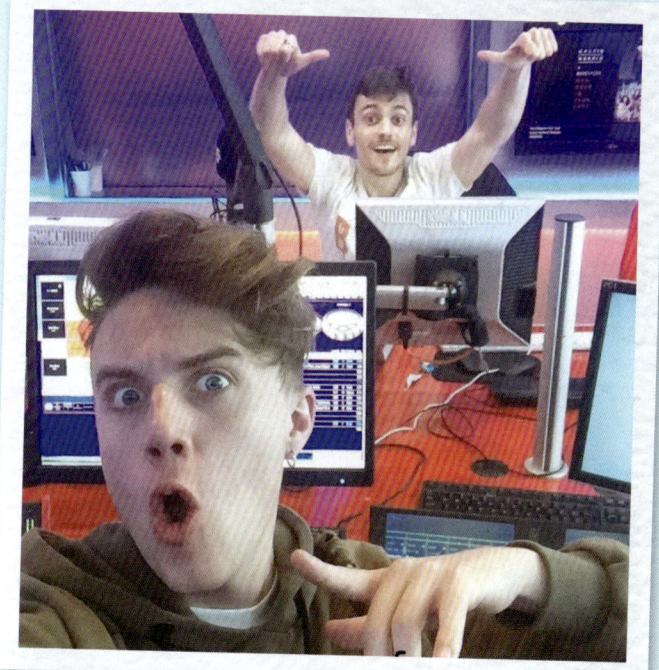

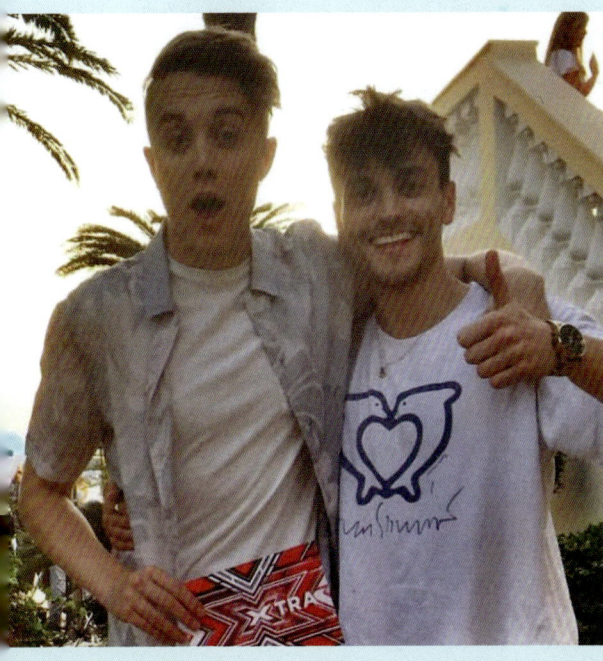

Joe was always cool and I wanted to be his friend from the start. Soon we went from being work colleagues into genuine mates

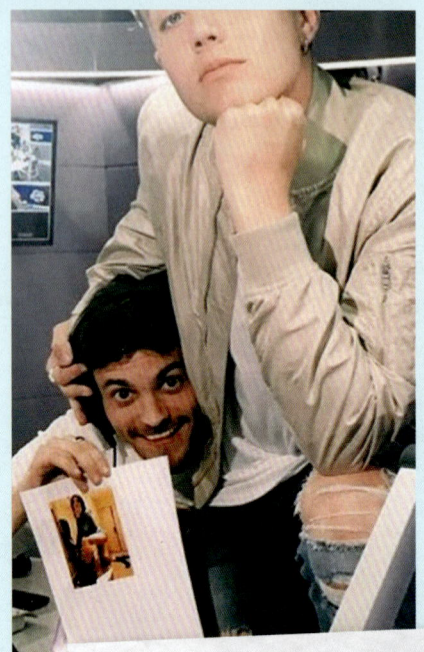
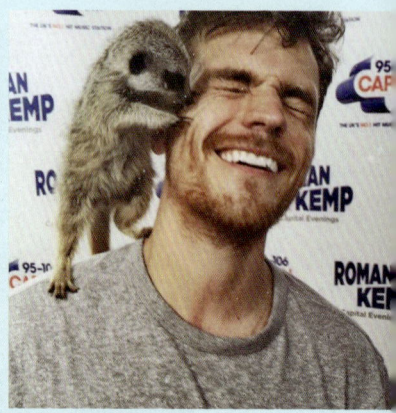

Here's a pic of Joe with a meerkat on his shoulder! We did so many crazy things. We were a double act and so close – I felt like he was the older brother I never had

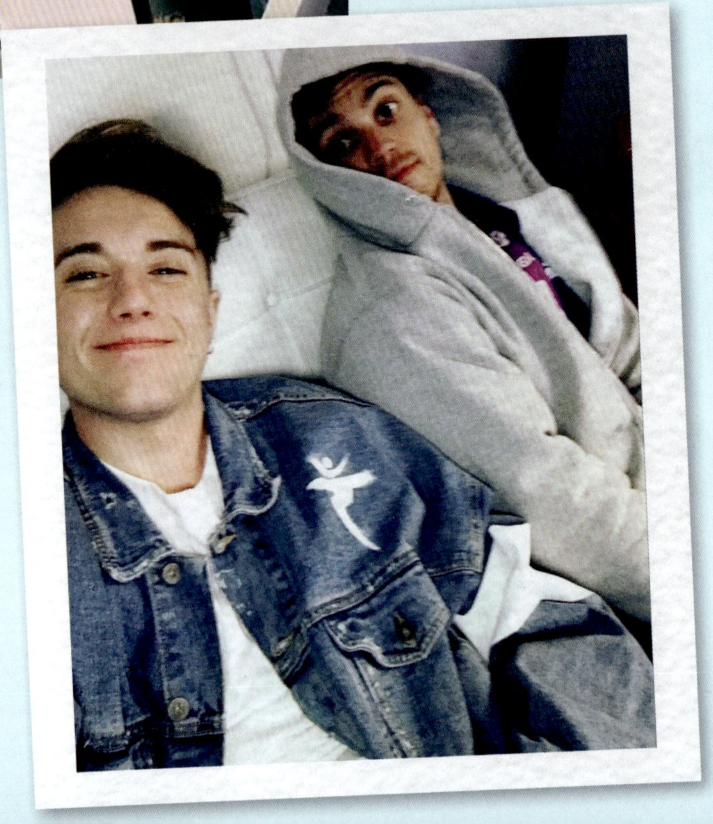

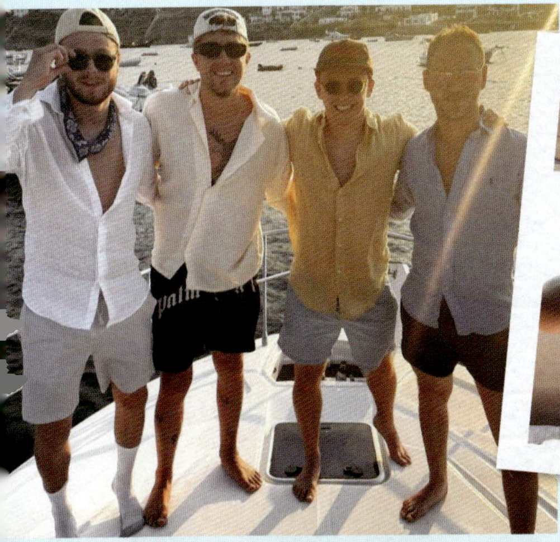

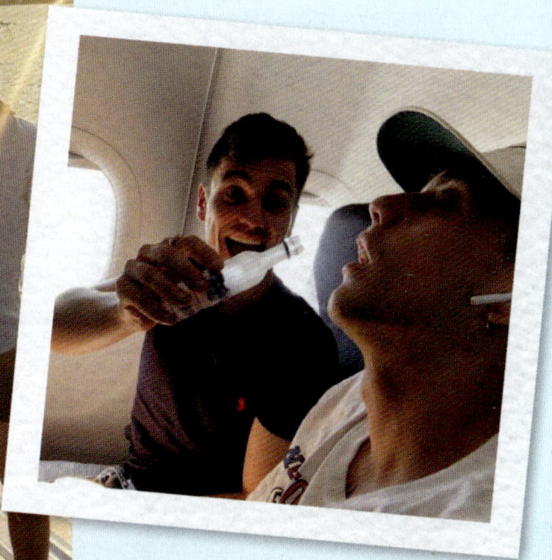

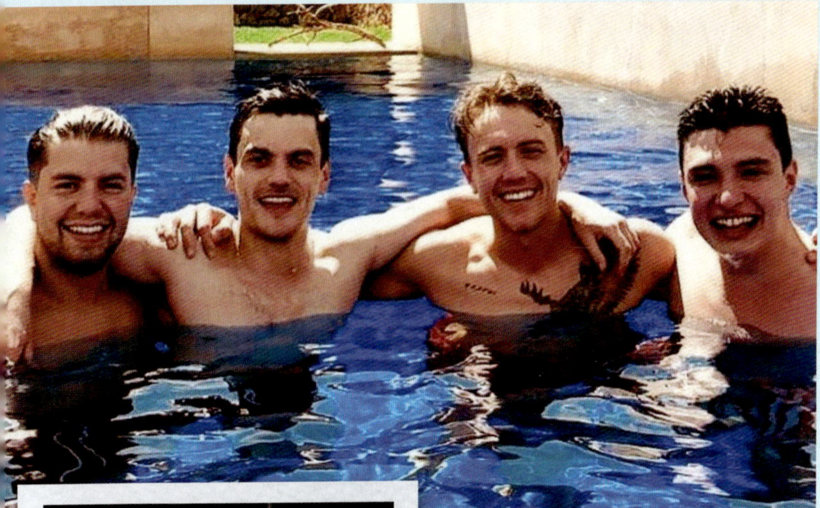

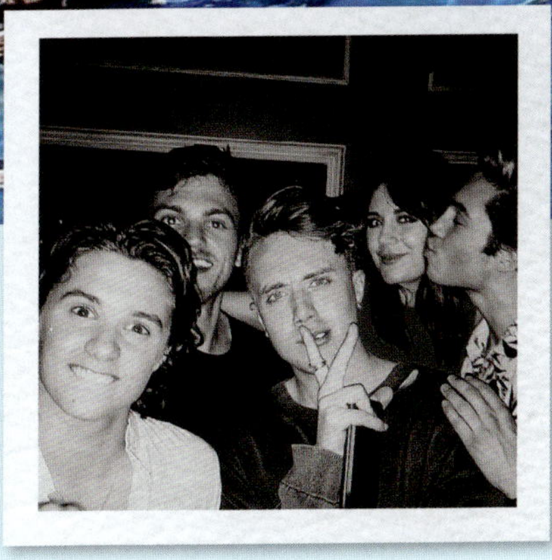

Happy holidays. Another page of pictures involving Joe. One of the many reasons why I was so angry at him, after he'd gone, was because he never spoke to me about just how he was feeling. There was never any inkling that anything could be so badly wrong

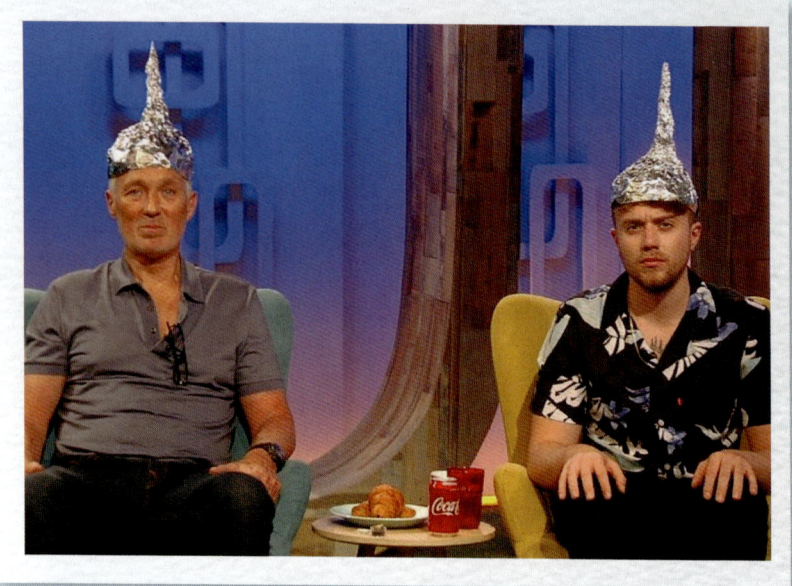

Acting daft with Dad on our 'Weekend Best' show. It was interesting because for the first time the roles had changed, Dad wasn't a presenter and I was suddenly coaching him how to do things. Like how he could ad-lib a bit to be less robotic!

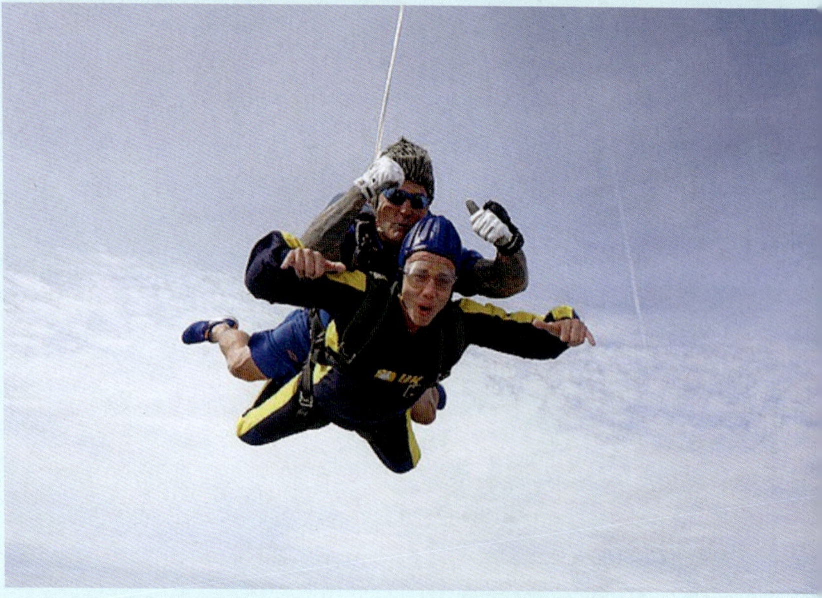

I'd fall for you. What an experience this was – getting the opportunity to try a skydive

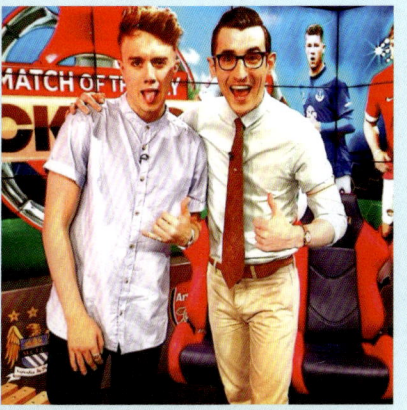
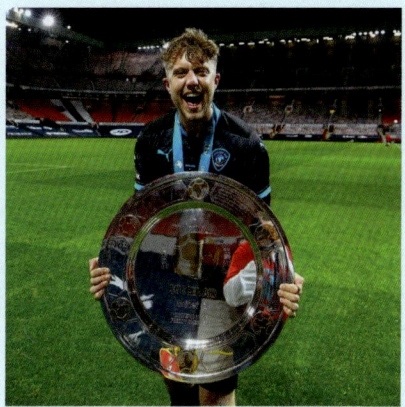
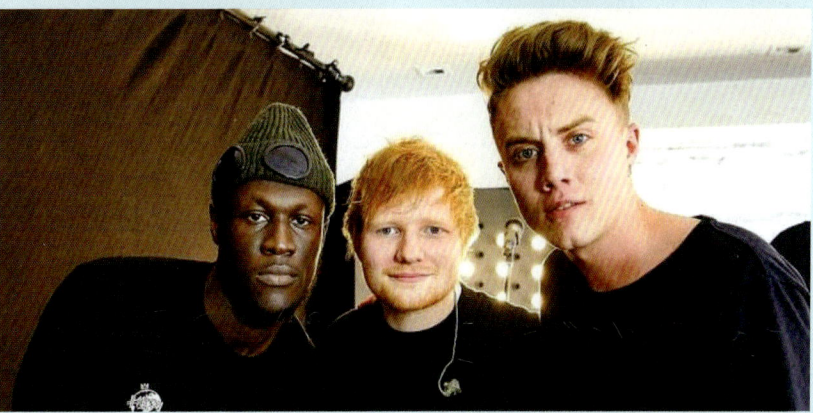
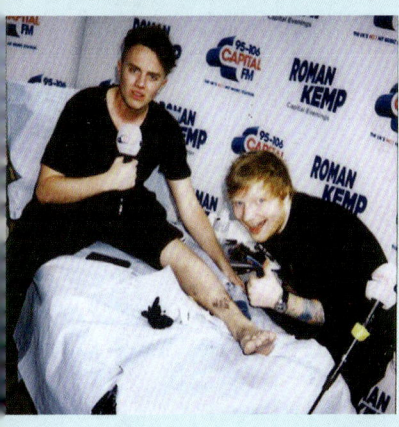
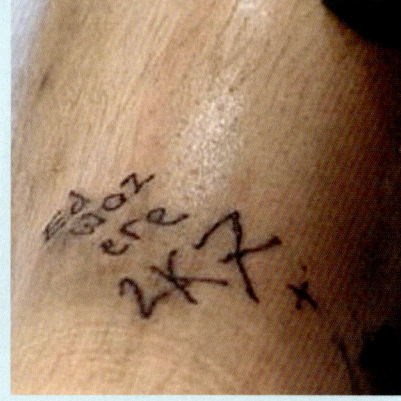

Famous mates. *(Clockwise from top left)* getting a footy buzz as a guest on Match of the Day Kickabout; celebrating a Rest of the World win at Soccer Aid (check out my dual passport!) and with Stormzy and Ed Sheeran – who tattooed my leg with a classy message, ha ha

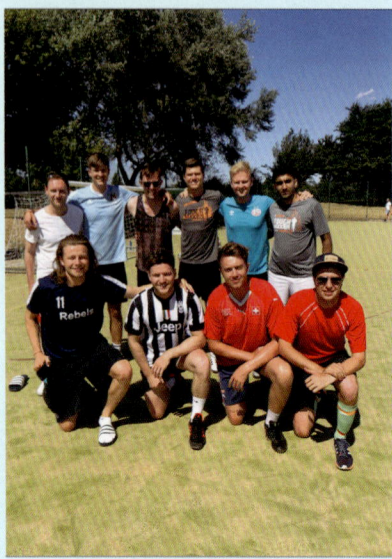

Netflix and Skill... Wednesday nights are sacred to me. I've turned down dates and good money for jobs, all because I don't want to miss my weekly kickabout. Here's a pic of me with my team Bedmond Ajax on a footy trip abroad

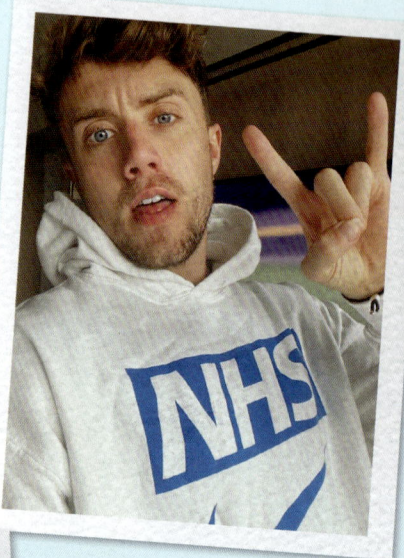

Big up to the nurses and doctors. Lockdown taught us all who the real heroes are. The NHS clapping was very moving

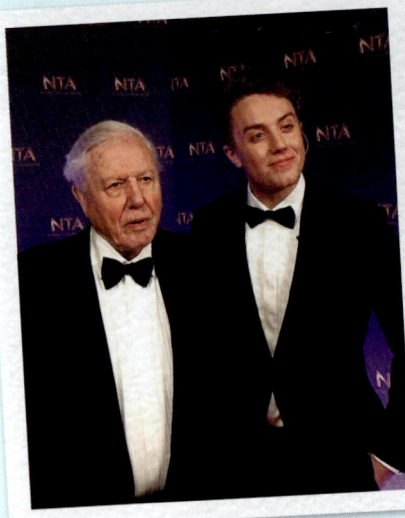

I hope that the great Sir David Attenborough approved of my impression of him on national telly!

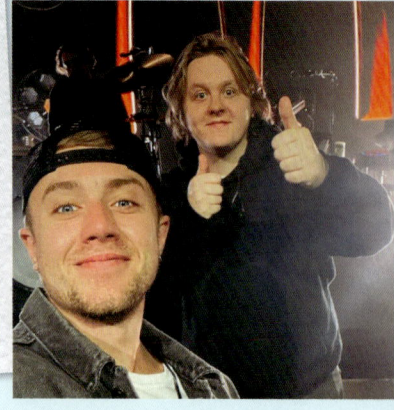

Another night out? Oh go on then... Lewis Capaldi is a top bloke and we often go to an 'old man' pub together

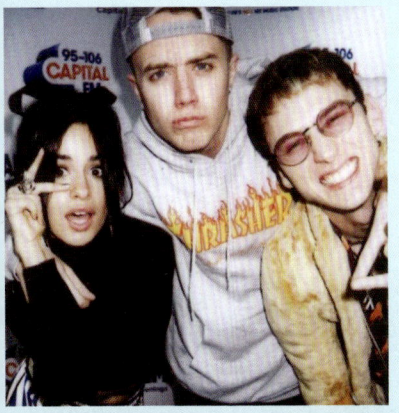
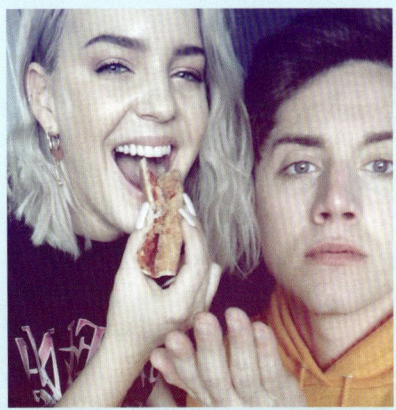
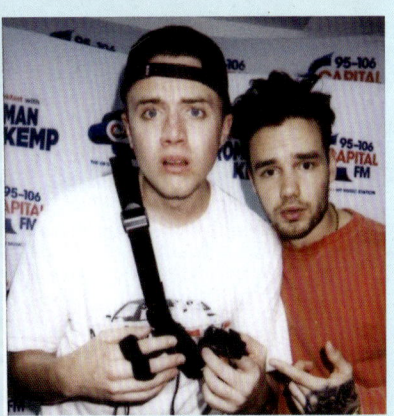
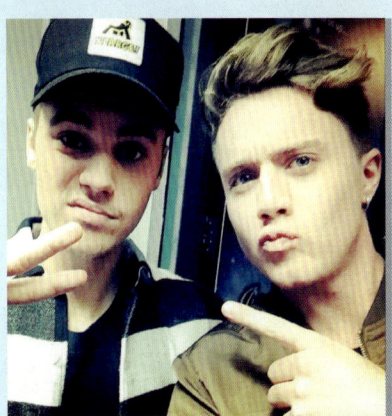
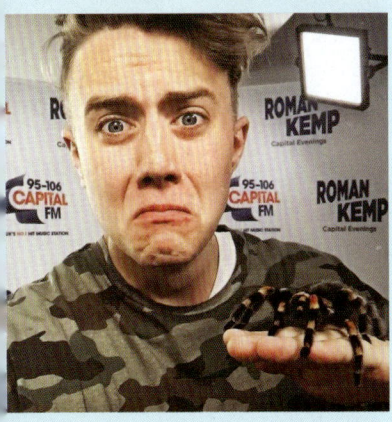
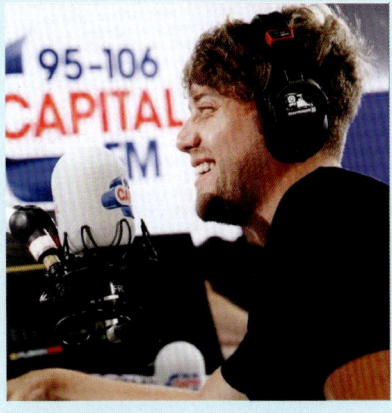

Capital gains. I've had some amazing experiences in my radio job and met so many amazing guests. Pictured here are me with Camila Cabello and Machine Gun Kelly; Anne-Marie; Justin Bieber – I've had some fun times with him – and Liam Payne

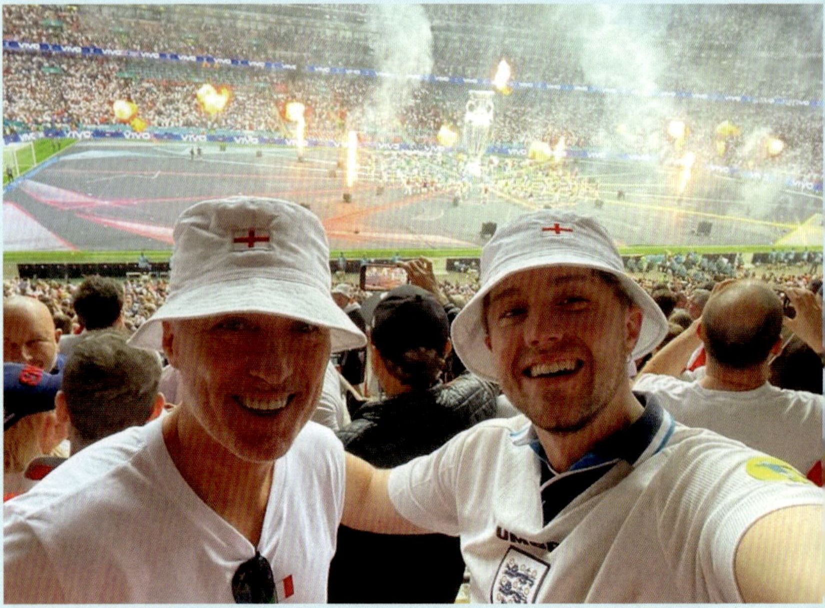

I took my dad to the football final of Euro 2020 at Wembley – I knew it would be the best present I could get him for his 60th birthday. We had England shirts and bucket hats on and it was amazing – an experience we shared that we will always remember

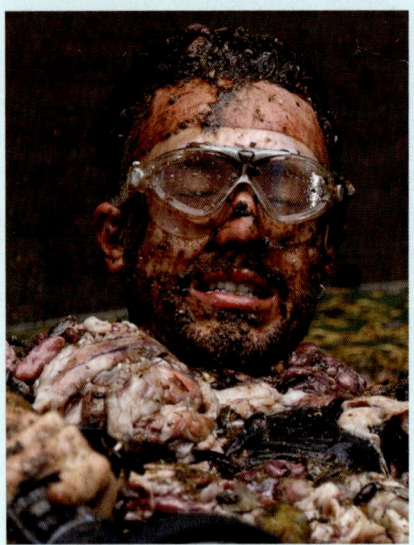

Believe it or not, going into the jungle was one of the happiest times of my life. It all felt so beautifully simple and I could be myself

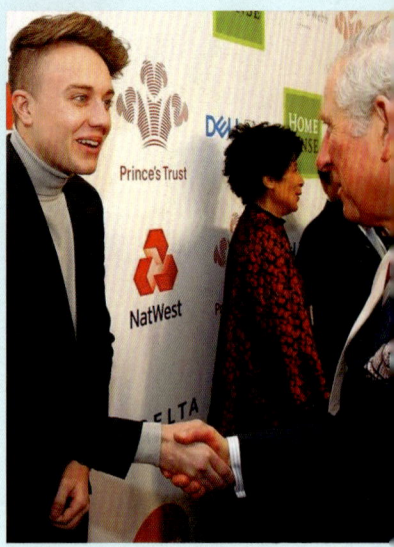

I really love the royal family. Here I am shaking hands with Prince Charles – now King Charles III of course

THE BIG LIST OF MY LIFE

HOLIDAYS

'We raised toasts to Joe, and recalled all the funny stories over the years, and it felt like he would approve. It was one of the best holidays I've ever had'

It's fair to say that I LOVE going on holiday. That's when I'm at my very happiest. Getting out of London, switching off from work, escaping demands, being able to sleep. Discovering new things, food, ways of life and people. I love being able to break away from the routine and feeling genuinely free and alive. Complete heaven. I go on holiday to fantasise about a different way of life that I might have when I'm older.

Getting on a boat is simply the best thing I can think of – that's when I feel at my most free and the tension lifting from my shoulders. Away from all the stress. No one can bother you on a boat. Perhaps that's why George Michael loved them, too.

I have a recurring fantasy of either being back in the jungle or on a boat sailing around the world. I just love, love, love being away from it all and having the chance to get a better perspective on life. Going to places like LA is my idea of hell, you feel like you're trapped in a bubble in those places, where everything is about how you look or what you're achieving.

I went to Jamaica in February and it struck me how simple life was there. The people have comparatively little to what we have in the UK, it's not about flashy cars and fashion and owning stuff. And yet they seem like they're the happiest people on Earth who have reached the perfect level of contentment just living their lives. I constantly fantasise about not living in the UK, no one caring who I am or what I have to do, who I have to meet or what I need to wear.

I always worry I'm the most boring holiday companion on Earth, because I get so much fun through my working life and what I do for my job, when I go on holiday I want to do almost nothing. Watch movies on Netflix. Eat nice food. And sleep a lot!

What I most enjoy is being away from all the noise and all the expectations that can affect my mental health.

I never want to moan about being in the public eye. But if I go somewhere where no one recognises me, it means no one will ask for my picture.

Sometimes, if I'm having a bad day, even something as simple as being asked for a selfie can make me feel bad. It's not about avoiding pictures and attention because you find it annoying or you're irritated by the person asking. But if you're having a bad day in your head it can be hard to deal with. Maybe you're having a day where you don't feel like you look particularly good, or you're just not feeling happy and worried that if that one photo comes out and you look unhappy then people will say, 'Oh, that guy's a dick,' you know?

So the reason I always say yes to photos is because I'm always so scared that someone is gonna go away and think I am a twat. Not being faced with that situation just feels more relaxing.

I can get recognised in funny places.

In April I went on a trip with my mum for her 60th, where we drove around the middle of the desert in America. We ended up in this little truck stop and someone came up to me and asked for a photo. How the hell they have ever listened to Capital out there, I'll never know. But it was funny. I love the work I do, and if being in the public eye is part of that I'll do it. But being famous is not what I chase.

I think the reason many celebrities seem to like going to Dubai is because there's a law that people can't take photos of you. Seeing bad pictures of yourself on the beach is never going to do much for your self-esteem, is it?

I've started trying to rent a villa every year in Mykonos, one of the Greek islands, where I say to all of my mates – just get your own flights, come and join me and I'll cover everything else. What's the point of earning decent money unless it's to do fun things and spend time with the people you really love? And the people who let you be who you really are? That's definitely a lesson I learned from Yog. I just like us all to be together so I can say thank you to them for being there. We'll sit around for hours chatting about everything. There's no pressure to 'perform', it's a chance to properly chill.

We did that after Joe died.

Joe was supposed to be on that holiday too, two weeks after he died. We wondered before if it was right to still go, but we decided it was important to be together and I invited the Capital lot to that too. We raised toasts to Joe, and recalled all the funny stories over the years, and it felt like he would approve. It was one of the best holidays I've ever had.

Going on holiday will always be a priority for me. But I have to admit I start getting the dreads – about returning to reality – as soon as I'm on the plane home. The thing I most dread is returning to the judgement and expectations on me I feel I have waiting for me at home.

Places I Love To Remember...

My favourite places in life aren't smart restaurants or clubs or anywhere people would want to Instagram really – they are the places where I have felt at my happiest. And being able to return to them, even just in my head, makes me feel calm inside.

Gillespie Road
Being taken to the original Arsenal stadium for the first time as a young kid will always stay with me. The greenness of the grass, the sheer scale of the pitch, the complete buzz of the fans. The smell of fried onions from the burger stalls always takes me back to that first memory of holding Dad's hand in my little football strip.

I watch as many games as I can at the Emirates Stadium. But the old one has a special place in my heart.

The Caribbean
Yes alright, it sounds a bit bougie of me saying the Caribbean, I know. But it's not because it's picture perfect, it's just such a different way of life. And it gives me perspective to say to myself, 'Look, if all else fails, you can go here.' The people are living their life simply and slowly, and it's beautiful. There will be stresses, of course. But walking in the sand, watching the sun set, and soaking up the chilled vibe makes everything seem right in my head.

There's a lot to be said for paring life right back to the basics, like I did in the jungle.

Chorleywood Common
I love going back to see my parents, but they've moved house

since I've left home, so I don't have that connection and longing for their home.

But Chorleywood Common was always where I'd come to walk the dogs with Mum as a teenager. Again, it was her theory that guys communicate better when you're not looking directly at them, so she'd often drag me off for long dog walks around the common near where they lived in Hertfordshire.

It's a beautiful green space and makes me feel calm being surrounded by trees and seeing the dogs run around. I still head up when I want to escape all the business of London. You can walk and not bump into anyone else. And when we made the BBC3 documentary, Our Silent Emergency, I brought Mum back up here when I needed to have an emotional chat with her and admit I had considered taking my own life.

It felt a safe place to talk because we've spent so many times walking and talking together here.

And Places I Want to Forget...

There are some places just make me feel sad inside.

Showbiz parties and the red carpet

I've never really liked parties. Hanging out with mates is nice. But parties or corporate events are my idea of hell. Any work sort of bash where you're expected to network – ughhh! I hate all that bullshit, and my PR team despair of me because I'm so reluctant to engage in it. The red carpet is like a cattle market and makes my skin crawl.

Ladbroke Grove, west London

There's nothing wrong with the area itself, only my associations with it. When I was 18 and modelling I was walking around the streets of Ladbroke Grove wearing a backpack with my portfolio, wallet, keys and phone. A couple of lads on bikes stopped in front of me. Some shouted at me from behind, I turned around and got punched straight in the face, then they took my bag. It wasn't so much that I was scared, it was more inconvenient, at a time when I was fairly unhappy.

Upstairs at Nan's house
Seeing inside Mum's parents' bedroom made me realise for the first time that a couple can be together and yet despise each other. Their room had two separate, single beds which seemed so lonely and symbolic of their bad relationship. Divorce isn't necessarily something that should be feared. It's something that should be spoken about. But I remember that room and shudder at the unhappiness that lived there.

The headmistress' office
It was never good if you got sent there at school. I remember once having to go and eat my peanut butter sandwich all by myself in her room and feeling particularly horrible.

Sainsbury's checkout
The supermarket where I got my bank card declined when I was trying to buy a meal deal…!

THE BIG LIST OF MY LIFE

CARS AND TRAVEL

***"I've killed someone,' I sobbed, words all
jumbled... Panic was flooding me'***

You'll never see me post on social media bragging about my car, that kind of toxic masculinity vibe is not my bag at all. I do like a nice car but it's only recently I've got myself one. This is entirely because Mum and Dad have warned me so many times over the years not to waste my money!

As soon as I was 17, I couldn't wait to learn how to drive. I failed my first driving test for speeding and I was gutted, but I immediately put in for another one and passing that second time felt fantastic. But it turned out to be a day I will never forget...

Vauxhall Corsa
My very first car was a little black Vauxhall Corsa. I had some money from the band, and some money from Dad, and I couldn't have felt prouder getting behind that wheel. I passed the test at 8 o'clock in the morning, and I spent the whole day driving. I was that excited, I went to Charlie's house, Matt's house, happily showing off my newfound freedom in my brand-new wheels.

In the evening I drove out to my then girlfriend's house in Buckinghamshire, I picked her up and we went to Zizzi's for a celebratory dinner. Going to any restaurant that didn't have pictures of the food on the menu felt very bougie back then! I didn't drink any alcohol, I've always been strict about not drinking and driving, and why would I need any booze? I was high on life.

After eating it was dark outside and we headed back to the car. Winding through the country roads was always slow progress as you had to keep pulling to one side to let other cars pass.

I certainly was under the speed limit. But all of a sudden the hedge to my left hand side just vanished and there seemed to be a car dazzling headlights instead.

What I hadn't realised was – we'd crossed a T junction.

My girlfriend screamed 'Oh shit!' as a car coming about 50mph slammed into the side of our car, lifting us up onto two wheels. The airbags went off, covering us with dust and there was glass and smoke everywhere.

Then silence. I remember my body going into shock. I couldn't understand what was going on. I looked over at my girlfriend – she was OK, thank God – but her door was jammed. Terrified, I knew we had to get out. I pulled her over from the passenger side and we somehow scrambled out the car to safety.

My main fear and dread was what had I done to the other person? I looked over and this man was in his car, eyes closed, and the front was completely crumpled. There were two cars behind him, and the people from those had got out and were trying to help him.

Have I killed someone?

It was my fault and I'd driven over a Give Way. I was so, so scared in those seconds.

I rang Dad. 'I've killed someone,' I sobbed, words all jumbled. 'I've killed someone, you're going to kill me, just kill me now.'

Dad was calm, asking whether I was hurt, asking whether my girlfriend was hurt.

Panic was flooding me.

Then the man in the other car opened his eyes, and he got out of the vehicle. I think I fell to my knees in relief and cried some more.

As it turned out, the man in the car was an ex-police officer who knew that that road was one of the biggest blackspots in the area. He was incredibly understanding. In the weeks that followed, as we went through the insurance and the police procedures, I certainly did a lot of growing up.

Everyone, including my girlfriend, could see it wasn't reckless driving on my behalf. But it was a mistake. And it was a real wake-up call to adult life.

It gave me flashbacks and nightmares in which I would be re-tracing all my steps from leaving the restaurant to the accident. Ultimately, no one was hurt and that incident made me a better and more careful driver. But I felt utterly shit that I'd endangered people's lives and my girlfriend's. It was my first brush with the police.

Eventually, I had that Corsa rebuilt. But it was a year before I got back behind the driving wheel again. My insurance jumped up to four grand a year after that. And thankfully I've never been in an accident since then. I'm so cautious now I've never even got a speeding ticket.

Mini Cooper
For a while I didn't have a car. But by the time I was 22 I'd moved out of home and was living in south London for a bit and decided I needed a little runaround.

So the next car I got was a little black Mini Cooper, Harley had a similar one so I thought it was a safe little car. Of course I would have secretly liked something a bit more flash, but I didn't feel I should spend any more, and Mum and Dad wouldn't have approved…

After a while though, I realised that cars in London can be a pain. Getting the Tube was easier. So I gave her up.

Mercedes G Wagon

By 2020, we were coming out of that first lockdown and I was missing being able to zip about under my own steam. I thought about getting a little cheap one, and then I thought, 'Nah, I'll treat myself to the dream car I actually want.'

So that's what I did! I've now got a matt black Mercedes G Wagon, which is great.

I think my parents realised I've worked hard for it, but I did a little sales pitch to them anyway to show I'd thought about it and wanted it and wasn't splashing out on a whim. I did let myself feel a bit proud getting it, you know, like I might be doing something right, and it's OK to let yourself enjoy life a bit.

And other ways I get around…

One of my favourite ways of travelling around London is by foot. When I was modelling I would get off the Metropolitan line from the suburbs, then trek around the city with my casting book with my headphones on being in my own little world. I feel like I know the city streets better than a London cabbie because of that time. Walking was my way of getting my cardio exercise in, and the streets of London never fail to inspire me.

THE BIG LIST OF MY LIFE

This is slightly embarrassing to admit, but I only learned to ride a bike in my 20s when I went on holiday with a girlfriend! As a kid I did have a bike, but I was more into skateboarding or rollerblading. I also got into ice skating when I played ice hockey at Ally Pally.

During the pandemic I bought my first proper bike and started cycling into work, which I still sometimes do now.

I went from being a nervous flyer as a kid to becoming a frequent one. At some points in my career I was catching planes more than once a week, so that quickly got me over my fears. The first time I started making some good money in my early 20s I treated myself to flying first-class for a long haul flight to America.

I sat down feeling pretty happy with myself in one of those big plush seats, only for the airline steward to come and ask me if I was lost and was I sure I was sitting in the right seat!

I didn't take offence, but stuff like that pushes me to prove myself sometimes.

If I want to fly first-class or business now, I don't feel guilty. Why should I? Well, within reason! I want to be as comfortable as possible and to get some sleep, so if it's an investment in myself for the right reasons then I feel I can justify it. The holiday starts as soon as you're on the plane as far as I'm concerned.

HOME

'I remember Mum was so kind after I'd just moved in and was having a bit of a tough time mentally'

Research has shown that your environment can really have a strong impact on your mental health.

Safe, comfortable and relaxed – this is how everyone wants to feel in their own home, right? I like to know I have somewhere I can retreat to escape the rest of the world at times.

Your home environment is where all your thoughts first start, and I know I feel more positive if I'm sat in mine and I can look around and see it's clean and clutter-free. So I am a bit of a clean freak and it just makes me feel calmer, more organised and more in control of life generally when things are tidy.

I always know immediately if I go round to a mate's house and it's really messy, they're no doubt having a bit of a messy time mentally.

Having a good old declutter – giving away to charity the stuff you don't need – does wonders for your state of mind. I find it genuinely therapeutic.

I truly believe that certain objects can hold so much power over you mentally if they've got meaning attached to them. When I've broken up with girlfriends in the past, I've just had to be ruthless and just chuck stuff away that reminds me of them because I don't want to see things and think about times that will put me in a bad headspace.

Even at my age, I still love my mum coming over and bringing candles or bed sheets washed in a familiar washing powder. Sounds ridiculous, I know, but if these small things can improve how you feel, they're worth doing, right?

I've lived in different places over the years, and each of them have had an impact on how I felt at the time.

Highgate, Hampstead Lane

While I was born in LA and we spent my first three years there, we always had our home in Highgate. It was a tall Victorian townhouse with a pretty walled garden. I remember having my very first birthday and the teddy bear's picnic cake and our Doberman Emma looming over me. We had a Donald Duck teapot which only came out for birthday parties.

This was the house where Dad was poorly, so there were some sad times, but it's mainly happy memories I have here of feeling safe and secure. Yog lived locally so he was always around the house.

Muswell Hill, Ellington Road

After Dad was poorly and we had financial difficulties, we moved to a slightly smaller and less pretty house in Muswell Hill. But alongside bad things come good – and we made some lovely friends with our neighbours, who were a great support to Mum. They had a boy called Joe the same age as Harley, and a girl called Lily the same age as me. I played football with Lily the other week, so we're all still mates.

I remember being able to look out of the top of my window – we used to have a skylight in the attic – and being able to see the flashing light on top of the pointy Canary Wharf office tower block. Dad told me it was a lighthouse.

I remember getting my first PlayStation in this house, and I would play football locally at Ally Pally each Saturday as well as going to the summer football camps every year. My bedroom was everything Batman here.

Rickmansworth, Hertfordshire
When Dad got the job in EastEnders we moved out to the sticks. I think Mum was sick of all the stairs in the London houses, and the traffic, and we had a modern house with wide rooms. I remember feeling slightly weird going from being a city boy to being surrounded by trees, and Mum says she regretted it as soon as we moved in! But I was football crazy so loved having a big garden to kick the ball in, and I had an Arsenal duvet cover.

We moved to another house, a much bigger one, in the same area after four years, where I spent my teen years. I painted my bedroom all black, and I had a big leather chair shaped like a baseball glove that swivelled around. I was so proud of that chair I got it for Christmas one year! We had a games room downstairs, our own space, where Mum and Dad let us have discos, parties and mates over all the time.

When Harley and I left home, Mum and Dad moved to a smaller place. And now they're building their own kind of dream home, which I am so proud of them for as it's long been their ambition.

Angel, north London
I was about 18 when I moved out and started renting a flat. It felt so cool to have a key to a flat. I couldn't get my head around how people remembered their keys all the time though!

THE BIG LIST OF MY LIFE

Dalston, east London
It was my breaking out years. I moved in with a girlfriend for the first time, here I was a fully grown-up man! With a car and flat. Or so I thought at the time…

Brixton, south London
The very place where Mum and Dad were worried about me hanging out as a teen ended up being the first place I actually bought. I was the first person in the family ever to move south of the river.

I remember Mum was so kind after I'd just moved in and was having a bit of a tough time mentally. I didn't have much furniture and I walked in the door and Mum had set it all up for me and made it like home with a light and bedding that smelt like home. It meant so much – she gave me a big hug and just told me that she loved me. It really pulled me out of a bad place and made me feel settled.

Vauxhall, south London
I love the two-bed flat where I live now. It's easy to get to work and I get a view of the city. Mum and Dad have a little place nearby for when they're in town.

FAME

'There are times when being in the shadow of famous parents left me feeling insecure and questioning my own self-worth'

I can't remember a time when I wasn't aware my dad wasn't famous. Even when I was little I'd always be able to clock people looking at him, whether we were at a football match, a restaurant, or just walking down the street.

People often ask how that affected me growing up, and in truth it's a difficult question to answer, because I don't have anything to compare it to.

There are times when I've loved it. When I was little I'd sometimes revel in the extra attention we'd get, and I'd enjoy showing off that my dad was Steve Owen in EastEnders. We didn't go to many celebrity parties, but I remember being taken to Liam Gallagher's house one time, and I thought that was very cool. Not because I knew much about Oasis back then, but because Liam gave me some Star Wars toys! But there are also times when being in the shadow of famous parents left me feeling insecure and questioning my own self-worth.

Even from a young age I felt a bit 'different' at school, I wondered if other kids were only friends with me because of who my parents were. If I got invited to parties and things like that, I wondered if it was because other kids' parents wanted to get to know mine. Or I became self-conscious about them talking behind my back.

I could see there was a slightly different atmosphere at the school gates when Mum and Dad turned up. And in some ways I loved it because I was so proud of them, but it certainly made me a little wary, too. Dad and Harley are pure sunshine and see the best in everyone, but I think Mum and I can take a little longer to trust, we tend to gauge people's motives a bit more.

Mum says she spent a large part of the 1980s hiding under a hat and sunglasses! She reckons that was all the rage back then. She saw up close the negative effects that massive fame had on George Michael. How he'd become something of a recluse. I remember constantly seeing Mum upset about how it all mentally affected Yog. She felt like she had lost her friend to this fucked-up 'fame beast'. It served as a real warning to me that chasing fame doesn't lead to nice places.

Because I'm so insanely proud of Dad and Mum's achievements in life, they are hands down my ultimate heroes, I will never moan about growing up in their shadow as I wouldn't want to detract from their success.

Dad is amazing at handling being in the spotlight. He always makes an effort to chat to people who approach him.

But he's also warned me that it's rude to just go up and take a selfie with someone and then walk off. I was often tempted to do this myself as a kid if I saw a famous footballer – but he told me not to. He's of the pre-selfie obsession generation and thinks you should just live in that moment and enjoy seeing someone you like or admire with your own eyes.

If you really want to make their day, he says, tell them you've appreciated something they've done rather than meaningless selfie-taking. He thinks that's more polite, especially if you're invading someone's private dinner. Not just waving a phone in their face and then sodding off after the picture's been taken. I can see his point.

I've also learned from him that it's not always easy being in the company of someone famous.

I spent a large time growing up with Dad being the person who would get handed a camera by a fan and asked if I could take a picture for them. I cringe a bit now when my friends get this treatment when they're with me because I know how that feels. I never want a partner to feel like this when they're with me, I can't stand the idea of them feeling like second fiddle in the way my mum sometimes was.

But Dad is always polite and respectful towards everyone and I've learned a lot about fame from watching him over the years. You'll never hear him moan, he's taught me that if someone says something you don't like, or does something that upsets you – like a girl you're on a date with tips off the paparazzi when you're out – your best bet is to shrug it off.

If you're going to be on a TV show that is watched by millions of people, he insists, you're sticking your head above the parapet, and you can't expect to not get hit sometimes.

'And what?' is what Dad often says. Meaning – has it ruined your life? Of course not – so shut up, be grateful for what you have, and move on.

Pros and cons of being famous

There are positives and negatives in doing a job where you get recognised. The good part is that we get to do fun stuff and speak to interesting people. The con is that when you're out for dinner, someone may want to keep looking over and come and interrupt you. More recently, I have had people come up and want to talk to me about suicide, and I don't always want to be reminded of losing Joe. Some days I genuinely feel he's cursed me with this mantle! But I know if I can be of any help I will always try and listen. It's too important not to.

The idea of being famous for simply being the son of someone famous was a horrific, hideous concept for me. I loathed the idea of someone thinking I've got where I have for coasting on my parents' coattails. The reason I turned down I'm A Celebrity the first time I was asked on the show was because I knew this would be how I'd be seen. It was only after I felt I had put in enough effort to achieve something myself in my own career that I felt ready to expose my 'real self' in the way that show demands you to.

And weirdly, as I've explained, spending time in the jungle entirely changed my mentality. The sheer simplicity of jungle life was something I'd never experienced before. It made me realise that fame is all a load of shit. Being able to go to a nice restaurant? Being able to wear the nicest clothes? Being able to drive nice cars? Really, it's all complete bullshit.

The happiest I've ever been was in that small little camp, wearing the same clothes every day that I had to hand wash myself, and eating a seriously limited diet – just enough to keep my body fuelled. It made me think that if it all goes wrong, then fuck it, I know how to live simply and I know the things that make me genuinely happy. Fame is not one of them.

When fame can be a pain

If I get the Tube to go to a gig or something and there's a large group of lads drinking, inevitably someone will spot me and start singing Spandau Ballet's hit Gold. Or shouting stuff about my parents.

Sounds harmless, I know, and don't get me wrong, I generally go unnoticed – I'm hardly Madonna! – but some days I just want to be left alone.

I went to a pub last week and was just minding my own business having a couple of beers with friends. Then a friend showed me that someone had secretly filmed me and posted it on their Instagram stories with the caption 'Roman Kemp – moody c*nt.' No one had come and chatted to me, they just decided to do that. Mainly, I can laugh about it, but if you're feeling a bit shit it's not especially nice.

When I was in Ibiza earlier this year, I was dancing on a balcony having a great time. Downstairs there was a girl, who was obviously drunk, shouting at me. I couldn't really work out what she was shouting, but eventually heard her say that she was a nurse and she wanted to talk to me about mental health. I was on holiday in the middle of a rave! I didn't want to just ignore her, so I said, 'Not now if you don't mind, let's talk later.'

Well, half an hour later she was in tears and trying to throw shit at me – cups and stuff – while her mates were trying to stop her. You know, I'm not saying anyone should feel sorry for me at all. But sometimes it's awkward.

Typical conversations when your dad is famous

This sounds ridiculous, but the following exchange happened recently, and it's what I hear a lot. I was knackered, feeling a bit crap and in a hurry while trying to collect my dry cleaning from the guy in the shop. It's not bad, I can't moan, I'm just telling you how it is.

THE BIG LIST OF MY LIFE

Me: Hi mate, here to collect stuff.
Him: What's your name?
Me: Roman.
Him: That's a funny name.
Me: Yeah. I know.
Him: So are you Martin's boy?
Me: Yeah.
Him: Martin's great, I love your dad.
Me: Yeah. He is.
Him: He's such a great actor. He's talented.
Me: Yeah.
Him: Have you got any talents?
Me: No, not really.
Him: Oh well, maybe you'll get them later?
(And I'm still standing there waiting for my clothes.)
Him: Your dad's a good-looking fella.
Me: Yeah.
Him: *(Looking me up and down disappointed.)* Oh well, maybe one day you'll grow into your looks, too.

You've got to laugh, but sometimes it's not exactly great for my self-esteem.

MY GODFATHER

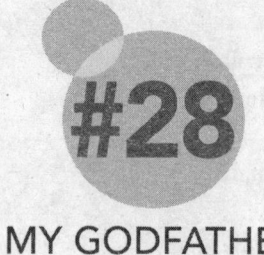

> *'Yog showed me what insane fame looks like – and why it's an ugly business...'*

I've never been fazed by meeting famous people in my life, because I grew up having George Michael as my Godfather.

You don't get a bigger name in showbiz than his. He and my mum were so close, more like siblings than mates, and George was very much an uncle figure to me and Harley throughout his life.

To us, he was never a world-famous pop star, or the best singer-songwriter of his generation, or an icon, or any of those other big labels bandied about. To us he was always just 'Yog'.

Mum was best friends with him long before he was famous, when they were both teenagers from the Watford area dreaming of success. He was always headed for stardom with all that insane talent he had, but Yog put in a lot of hard graft too to get Wham! off the ground.

Mum remembers them sitting together in his bedroom and sending off early demos of songs like Careless Whisper and Club Tropicana – and then getting them all, one by one, rejected. I'm sure many record labels were left kicking themselves about that after Wham! hit the big time.

Yog famously went on Mum and Dad's first ever date at the

THE BIG LIST OF MY LIFE

Camden Palace in 1983. Mum was so nervous she wanted Yog there as a chaperone, and Dad then spent most of the evening trying to get rid of Yog so he could make a move on Mum!

Yog was a huge part of all our lives.

Every summer holiday for as long as I can remember we went to his house in the South of France.

We'd catch a plane to Nice, and then Yog would arrange for a helicopter to pick us up from the airport and fly us to his house. It was the first time I'd ever got in a helicopter, my excitement as a kid was through the roof. Proper rockstar treatment! Having him so dominant in our lives taught me from a young age what that level of fame gets you in life… The good and, later, the bad.

He had a big old farmhouse, with a garage that had bats in, so Yog called it 'the bat cave' as I was so obsessed with Batman as a kid. I had the wallpaper, the duvet, the toothbrush, everything. And here I had my own bat cave too. Yog was always happy to indulge my imagination.

There was a lovely pool and we'd happily mess around for hours on his boat. I still love boats now thanks to those childhood memories. He had private chefs who cooked. It all sounds very bougie, I know. But it didn't feel especially flashy when we were there, it was just a lovely rustic villa and a place we could all really relax.

More than anything, Yog loved escaping that crazy fame side of his life and spending time with the people he loved.

Sometimes it would just be Mum, me and Harley. Sometimes Dad would come too, if he wasn't working. If Dad came he basically slept for the first two days. On a sun lounger, no sun tan lotion, he'd snooze away as he turned bright red.

One time, when I was about five, as the adults were busy chatting and Harley was playing backgammon with Dad,

I nearly drowned in Yog's pool. I'd taken my armbands off, and was messing around by the side of the steps with a truck, and the next thing I knew my right foot had given way and – SPLASH! – I was under the water, sinking straight to the bottom. I could see the underside of my inflatable crocodile at the top of the water and no one had noticed me and I couldn't breathe. I can remember the panic I felt as I struggled to get up to the surface.

After what felt like minutes, but was probably a matter of 30 seconds, Dad had spotted me and dived straight in to rescue me. When I came up coughing and spluttering he didn't tell me off. I imagine he felt pure relief. But I was marched straight into swimming lessons as soon as we got home!

There were never other families and kids at Yog's French house, so Harley and I would have the run of the place and access to Yog all to ourselves. It was carefree and brilliant.

Yog was a hugely caring person, if anyone needed help from him, they'd get it.

After Geri Halliwell left the Spice Girls in 1998, Yog took her under his wing. She was there one summer with us, and had her little Shih Tzu in tow. And while Dad was sleeping – and slowly turning the colour of a lobster – Harley brought him out a sandwich and put it on the table beside him.

When he didn't stir, Harley had the idea of letting Geri's dog nibble the insides of this sandwich. These things were always Harley's idea, but she'd enlist me to join in. So it was my job to bring over the dog and let it get at the meat, giving the bread a good old lick too. Then we re-assembled it, woke Dad up and told him lunch was ready.

He happily ate the whole thing before we told him what had happened. To be fair, Dad always took these pranks in good spirits. And Yog thought it was all hilarious, he had a great laugh on him, throwing his handsome head back and bearing those gorgeous white teeth.

Yog loved us, and having no kids of his own, he treated us like his family and could be very protective of us.

One of the biggest arguments I remember Mum and Yog ever having was when I was a teenager, around 14. Yog had come for dinner one night and the talk had turned to Mum's plans to move us all to LA. There were work opportunities for Dad there, he'd been offered some film roles, and I had an American passport. I imagine she just fancied a change of scene, raising us kids in the sunshine.

But Yog was adamant that this was a terrible idea, he was literally shouting at her because he thought it would have such a bad impact on me and Harley as teenagers. 'You will ruin your kids,' he yelled at her. 'You know what that lifestyle would do to them. They need to be as far away as possible from there, they need to have a normal life.'

They'd argued before, of course, but that was the biggest row I'd ever seen them have. And it ended up with George storming off in his car.

We didn't move to LA in the end.

I don't know how much of that decision was down to George persuading Mum it was wrong for teenagers to be exposed to LA life, but that's how fiercely protective of us he could be. And I didn't mind not going, I was happy at my school and with my mates.

Yog never spoke to me directly about fame. Or about mental health – neither mine nor his. People weren't so open. I know Mum saw Yog really struggle with his success – or rather the effects of his fame – throughout his life. But it wasn't something

I ever talked to him about. And Mum was keen to protect us from his more troubled side. As I grew older though, I could certainly see for myself his existence wasn't all dazzle and glamour and private choppers. He found that level of fame a dark and lonely place at times.

When you can't leave your own front door without being papped, and people are selling stories about you, of course you're going to have a lot more struggles mentally. About who to trust, about what is reality, who your real friends are, and all those types of things. It certainly gave me a strong distaste for people who want to be famous for the sake of being famous. I could see it wasn't what it was cracked up to be.

Over the years I'd witnessed how George was surrounded by people who always said 'yes' to him. And that's not good for anybody. If everyone always agrees with you, well… you quickly lose sense of what's real. What matters.

I think that's why he and Mum were always so close, he completely trusted her, and he also knew that she always spoke honestly to him, and argued with him at times. He needed and wanted that, instead of being surrounded by sycophants the whole time.

The thing with George is, people always assume he had this jet-setting lifestyle the whole time, but often he'd just come to our house and watch EastEnders hanging out with my nan, who he adored. More often than not, Yog wouldn't be living it up celebrity-style, he'd be sitting in front of the telly watching shows like Deal Or No Deal.

He had such a huge heart and generous spirit that he watched someone lose quite a lot of money once on that show, and he felt so bad for them that he found that guy later and paid him the money!

He loved my mum so much, they were almost like boyfriend and girlfriend and constantly on the phone together. But she was careful not to share with us the darker times Yog was having. I think she just wanted to keep our image of him as a very happy one, right to the end.

He'd spoil us rotten on our birthdays. And we'd always see Yog on Boxing Day or always in the Christmas holidays week.

Yog would bring extravagant gifts for me and Harley, which could be awkward if they were better presents than Mum and Dad's! Dad bought me a bike one year – which was great, I know, right? Then Yog swanned in, and he'd been to Harrods and got me an electric car, and not just any electric car but a huge Batmobile one! I was in heaven but it was probably quite annoying for my parents to be upstaged.

Then, as I got older, the incredible wish-list toys got replaced by very generous Selfridges vouchers. We were very lucky kids, I know.

Yog never got involved in shaping my career but when I landed my first job in a band, when I was 15, he was proud and also asked his lawyers to look at the contract I'd been given to check everything was in order.

It was only later, after his death, that all his family and his friends told me that George would always go on about me to them, and that he'd proudly talk about me working at Capital, and would listen to my show.

It makes me happy that he saw me have some success because he'd seen all the hard work and setbacks I'd been through to get to where I am now.

I don't like to remember anything but the nice times with Yog. The happy memories. The special moments we shared.

I love the first Wham! album, Fantastic, and it's still an

album now that I'll be able to listen to, and enjoy, and feel proud of the fact that Mum was part of that with Yog.

Yog's songs are timeless, you can always listen to them and get something new. And the songs in life that appeal to me most are always the ones with stories attached and real emotions.

Yog explained to me once the story behind one of his songs, Nothing Looks The Same In The Light. He told me that it was about the first time he'd slept with a man, and how he felt like this boy meant everything to him, and then all of a sudden the next day, the boy was gone and that was it. The relationship was over.

I guess that was Yog's first real understanding of what a one night stand was. He came away from that life-changing experience and wrote that song. Every time I listen to it I remember Yog being so open about his feelings with me, and just how much soul that guy had.

The Christmas Day he died, in 2016, was such an utter shock and misery. He was just 53. Way too young to go. We were due to go to Yog's Goring-on-Thames house in Oxfordshire the very next day, for a Boxing Day get-together.

On Christmas Day we were watching a film at home, Mum, Dad, me and Harley, on the sofa. The phone was ringing.

'I'm not answering that, it's Christmas Day,' said Mum, crossly. We were happy in our little festive bubble, the four of us together. But it kept ringing and ringing and ringing…

Eventually, Mum went out of the room to pick it up.

Then I'll never forget the agonising scream she let out, I'd never heard her make that sound in my life.

What the fuck had happened?

Mum ran into the room, not even able to form proper words, and she collapsed on her knees in the middle of the floor with the phone on loudspeaker. She just cried, 'Yog's dead.' And Dad immediately burst into tears. Neither of them could talk. So Harley took the phone and spoke to Yog's sister on the other end of the line.

The rest of Christmas went on in a weird and horrible blur. We knew that this awful thing was all of a sudden going to be on every single news channel in the world, and then we sat sort of numbly waiting for it all to unfold on TV. That is not a normal way of dealing with grief, when you're waiting for the whole world to pick up on it. It seemed ridiculous and surreal that Yog was really gone.

It was a very strange experience grappling with losing this huge force in our lives, while watching this outpouring of shock and grief from people we didn't know unfold in the media at the same time.

Yog's funeral wasn't until the end of March. But in February, just weeks after his death, Yog's bandmates – Andrew Ridgeley, Mum and fellow bandmate Pepsi – got up on stage at the BRIT Awards to pay tribute to George's phenomenal career.

Mum was so brave speaking in public about this best friend she had loved for so long. She spoke about Yog's incredible generosity, he gave huge amounts to charity that no one even knew about during his lifetime. Mum couldn't help breaking down in tears at one point as she described how he'd been like a brother to her, and remembered his magical way with words. Then Chris Martin from Coldplay came on and sang one of Yog's hits, A Different Corner.

It was a very emotional evening. I was already working for Capital then, and was having to host a show backstage that night. But seeing Mum come on stage and well up with tears remembering Yog all got too much for me to carry on working.

ROMAN KEMP – ARE YOU REALLY OK?

I'll always be grateful to Marvin Humes for that time. He's a DJ at Capital too of course, but that night he was just there as a guest with his wife Rochelle. And he kindly stepped in and did the rest of the show for me that night.

I've never felt prouder of my Mum than getting up there on stage and talking to millions of people about her best mate.

When it came to me having to talk about the loss of my own best mate, Joe, only a few short years later, I remembered Mum doing that, and it gave me courage when I had to say on air how we had lost him.

When I think about George now, I try to do it from a place of pride in him rather than sadness. Mum's always encouraged me to think about how incredible it is that he touched so many people at different times in their lives.

I know she's right. But it's still odd to think about George Michael belonging to the masses in that way. To me he will remain my mum's best mate, and my special and much-beloved Godfather Yog.

THE BIG LIST OF MY LIFE

LOCKDOWN

'Incidences of mental health went through the roof... but if you were lucky enough not to have been affected, then I think it gave some people the chance to relax and have a sense of gratitude and put life into perspective'

When the first lockdown came in March 2020 it felt like the world was ending. Like the rest of the population, I had no idea what to expect. I was actually due to go on holiday for two weeks in the April. Obviously, I wasn't going to be actually going anywhere, but I was still tempted to take the time off.

It was one of the few times ever in my life when Dad told me what I shouldn't do – and he was adamant that I should be at work. He said that people were relying on me to turn up and entertain them in the morning, as I normally would. He got on the phone and told me, 'This is your duty, Ro, you've got to go and do this,' and he was dead right.

Now, I daren't claim anyone remotely relied on me – or listening to Capital – to help them through the pandemic! But Dad was right. If there was some small way I could show up and be responsible and help people feel more normal when the world seemed mad, then I should do it. If I could make one person laugh that day, or help make them feel in a routine, it would be worth it.

ROMAN KEMP – ARE YOU REALLY OK?

People look to the radio for comfort in tough times. I think all you can do is be as real as possible. I got a lot of texts throughout the day on the show from ambulance drivers or hospital workers, and it's very easy to forget you are talking to other people when you're sitting in a radio studio.

It was a scary time in my life, both personally and professionally. I admit I felt daunted trying to be an escape for so many people, but I wanted to show up and be an adult and try my best.

In the middle of it I had chats with Chris Moyles, Greg James and Johnny Vaughan, and they all said to be as honest as possible, to keep going, so I'm grateful to those very experienced guys for helping me out.

I am patriotic, and I love how everyone seemed to pull together more in those crazy months. It made me so proud. My grandad used to tell me about the war, about how people would step up to fly planes, and he always said you'd be surprised at people in those situations. There was that first weekend when we needed volunteers for the NHS, and something like 700,000 people stepped forward. Those moments bring a massive sense of pride not only to those people, but to the whole country. The NHS clapping was very moving.

Also, from a selfish point of view, working during the Covid outbreak was brilliant for giving me a sense of normality and allowing me to leave the house. Because I was also filming Gogglebox and Sunday Best it meant that I got to see Dad because it was work. I was fortunate because other people couldn't see their loved ones.

I know people watching Gogglebox were going, 'How come they get to see each other?' but because it was work that was ruled acceptable. We all know how confusing the rules were at times, but selfishly that was a benefit I was lucky enough to enjoy.

I had a relationship break-up during lockdown, and like everyone else I missed being with my family, seeing Mum and Harley. But compared to so many families we were incredibly lucky. So many people were isolated, unhappy and grieving loved ones. Incidences of mental health went through the roof, and it breaks my heart how kids were affected.

But in terms of having to stay at home, speaking personally, I bloody loved it most of the time! I'm a bit of a hermit anyway so I enjoyed having that pressure to go out taken away. If you wanted a weekend at home not doing anything then it was perfect. And I loved the fact that celebrities like Kylie Jenner weren't posting glamorous events on social media, they were suddenly all the more human as we knew they were doing the same thing as everyone else – staying at home in their tracksuits.

If you were lucky enough not to have been affected, then I think it gave some people the chance to relax and have a sense of gratitude and put life into perspective.

We became more grateful for the tiny things that actually matter the most, like being able to see grandparents, when those restrictions were lifted.

When the rules allowed us to meet in parks with friends and do things in the summer, one of the last happy memories I have is of playing football with Joe on Clapham Common. He was normally a terrible footballer, but that time he actually scored a hat-trick. Some days I like to think he went out on that high as it makes me smile.

#30

RADIO & BACK TO JOE

'Joe came with me into the studio. He didn't have to – producers usually stay at home, they're not always sat with the presenter – but by then we'd become a real team'

I was 23 when Capital started getting me involved. They weren't going to let me loose on anything big. But they just needed a roving reporter for a silly prank job which required me to go around Trafalgar Square, in the centre of town, asking members of the public to try a made-up product for a slot on the breakfast show. Of course I said, 'Yes please!' It sounded right up my street.

It was the autumn of 2015, and that's when I met Joe Lyons for the first time. He was four years older than me and already a producer for the radio station.

I knew nothing about radio, and I think he took one look at me – some over-confident kid in black skinny jeans, brand-new trainers and a Nike windbreaker top – and inwardly rolled his eyes. Joe clearly thought, 'Why the hell am I having to babysit this gobby little celebrity's kid?'

He had a Tottenham hat on, so that wound me up, a denim jacket with fake shearling, and a Comrex backpack – which transmits radio – with just a single microphone. He spoke like Del Boy and even lived in Peckham! I thought it all seemed an amateurish set-up. I dunno what I was expecting, but after my (admittedly limited thus far) experience of TV, I was thinking 'Where's the camera? Where's the glitz and glam?'

Our first exchange was about football. Joe seemed dismissive and was clearly keen to get the job done and sod off home for breakfast.

The task he set me up with was to take something that looked like a Pritt Stick, but was made of butter instead of glue, and oh so hilariously dubbed the 'butt stick'. He handed me that, plus some crappy bit of toast and a paper plate, and my challenge was to take it to people roving around, get them to taste it, eat it and then buy it.

I just said, 'Cool! Let's do it,' and Joe warmed to me a bit. I think he realised I was a bit of a cheeky chappy and I didn't take myself too seriously.

Luckily, I have no embarrassment filter whatsoever. I've never minded making a fool of myself, or putting myself in awkward situations, like I'd done in the bar for the football videos. So I threw myself into the task at hand – and we smashed it out the park in 15 minutes. Job done, in the can, thanks very much.

It was silly fun, which is my vibe, and I loved it. 'Let's get the funny.' That was always what Joe said.

That first time, Trafalgar Square was like my audition for Capital, I guess. I didn't hear anything for a week or so, and then I got a call: 'Do you want to start making some demos for a show?'

Of course I did!

They wanted to hear what my voice sounded like on radio.

I grew up listening to Capital FM, it was always the show for me. It was young and it was fun. So I was made up to be given this chance.

ROMAN KEMP – ARE YOU REALLY OK?

I was nervous because I wanted it so badly. But at the same time, I told myself they weren't letting me loose on live radio. I'd be reading off a script and no one would hear it, it would be like a fake show, to test me out.

I remember walking into the office to do the demo and seeing Joe sitting there, still looking like a dishevelled Del Boy Trotter.

The first demo went well – they wanted me to do a real show! It was 1am-3am on a Sunday night. Basically, the real graveyard slot, as you can imagine there weren't many listeners tuning in at that time, but I didn't care. I was overjoyed. And I was paired up with Joe to teach me the ropes.

I was enthusiastic and willing to learn. But Joe saw me as an annoying little puppy dog. 'Sit there,' he ordered, almost rolling his eyes. 'Read this. Do that.' All I had to do was speak between the songs for a couple of minutes. Try to make people laugh and fill out those moments somehow.

Radio works on playlists. They use focus groups to listen to the music and compile the lists based on people's opinions so they are in tune with what listeners want. If you tune in to Capital, you want to hear the biggest and most popular songs. It stands to reason that most people in Britain only really listen to the radio in 20-minute segments. They may be in their car travelling to work or the shops, picking the kids up from school or even listening while they're cooking the dinner or doing household tasks. Their favourite station should be like a familiar friend, always there for them.

Anyway, Joe was always the harshest critic for me.

The first time I said the line, 'Hello everyone, this is Roman Kemp and you're listening to Capital Radio,' Joe immediately stopped the recording.

'Why are you saying "everyone"?' he asked.

'Because I'm speaking to everyone!' I said.

And Joe patiently explained that when you're listening to the radio, you're often alone, you like to think it's YOU being talked to. Not thousands of others too. It's personal.

Chris Tarrant – who I think is an amazing DJ – used to sit with a tennis ball with a face drawn on it in the seat opposite him. Then he'd do the whole show delivering to that 'ball' person. Radio is about intimacy and building a relationship with listeners.

When my first show went out at 1am I was so excited. My parents were listening at home and I'd set an alarm to go and listen to it while sitting in my little car, the Vauxhall Corsa.

After a few weeks of recording the night shows they let me do it live. With Joe by my side I was learning quickly.

Joe proved to be an excellent teacher, and he was never shy of pulling me up on my mistakes: I said 'wow' too often. And I had a high-pitched laugh that needed to go.

'That's not good. Don't do that,' he'd say. But he could see I was quick and eager to learn. Even now it's Joe's voice I hear in my head, telling me what I've done wrong, how I could be better.

Joe had been to university at Leeds and he'd been making radio for years. He loved comedy and did stand-up himself, he was a real grafter.

Despite cultivating this Del Boy image, with a mockney accent, Joe was actually from Surrey, and probably one of the poshest friends I had. He was the kind of guy who could go out and cane it at the weekend, but he was always shit-hot at his job and very ambitious.

He was cool and I wanted to be Joe's friend from the start.

And soon we went from being work colleagues into genuine mates. 'Prick' we'd call each affectionately. Or worse. We were constantly taking the piss.

Within three weeks, Joe had me learning 'the buttons'. When you walk into a radio studio it looks like a spaceship, all these buttons and switches and faders and things that send you live, which seem terrifying.

The night before I had to 'do the buttons' for the first time I honestly didn't sleep at all. I was so anxious I had heart palpitations.

But Joe came with me into the studio. He didn't have to – producers usually stay at home, they're not always sat with the presenter – but by then we'd become a real team. And I picked it up quickly, bar the odd mistake, when Joe would smirk at me sitting two feet away to my left. I felt safe with him by my side, and he nurtured me and taught me everything he knew.

By the time it came to Christmas 2015, another opportunity came up to shine.

No one wants shifts at Christmas. Everyone wants to be with their family or to go on holiday. So the station said to us, 'There's two weeks to cover – which one do you want?'

Joe and I immediately said, 'Both of them!' And that year we worked Christmas Eve, Christmas Day, Boxing Day, New Year's Eve. And I absolutely loved it.

For me, it was a case of putting in the air miles.

Ed Sheeran describes it really well when he talks about songwriting. He says he's at the 'clearwater' part of his career, which makes sense to me. At the beginning of anything new, it's like you're running the tap in an old house and the water's coming out a horrible brown colour, it's dirty and rank. But if you just keep it coming out, keep it coming… it'll eventually run clear. That's how I saw it. The more I talked, the more I learned. The more you relax into it, the more you can just chat and feel relaxed.

Joe was constantly analysing me, correcting me, and I completely put all my trust in him. Yet the one thing I know I could do was make him laugh. And I would do anything for Joe to find me funny.

I was always happy to be the fall guy, acting like an idiot to make it funnier. Because if I'd made Joe cry with laughter then it would have been a good day.

####

'I think some feathers were ruffled as Joe and I had become a unit, we were the cool kids at the station, proving ourselves, and I think some people were jealous'

####

It was during those two weeks over Christmas when we really bonded. We'd record clips, make each other laugh, we had a system going. We were producer and presenter but also genuine friends.

I never needed to pretend a tennis ball was a person, because I always had Joe. And if he was laughing I was doing my job. Our humour was very slapstick, we'd get obsessed with silly YouTube videos of crabs walking from side to side and put music to it.

He took great pleasure putting me in awkward situations, like the time he took me to my first strip club that Christmas.

I think he was trying to be cool. But we turned up at Platinum Lace in Leicester Square with no money, we paid for no dances, and we felt totally out of place and left after 20 minutes!

Joe and I spent many evenings just getting dinner together at Nando's.

Most of our ideas for the show were formulated over half a chicken and chips. Talking about football, relationships and work.

He was a good-looking guy and always had some crazy dating stories.

Joe became mates with all my best mates and I secretly wanted him to marry Harley – they were exactly the same age. But Joe had high standards and always imagined he'd end up with a Victoria's Secret model.

Joe came to my parents' house for dinners all the time, he'd phone my mum for a chat sometimes, and was at all my birthdays. People adored him, and anything I was invited to, so was he. They always said, 'Will Joe be coming?' and he always was. He was almost like my boyfriend. One time when we were on an away job, there was a fuck-up with the booking and we had to share a bed. 'Oh God,' he moaned, when he realised I'd have to bunk up with him.

He was a keen footballer but absolutely terrible. And he was an equally bad motorbike rider – he came off once and was on crutches for weeks. He'd poke with his crutch if he could see I was slumping at work. 'Come on Kemp, wake up, make me some money!' We were such a double act and so close I felt like he was the older brother I never had.

We'd chat about the show, our careers and how we could get to the next step. We were both ambitious.

I set myself a goal – I wanted to be presenting the breakfast show within 10 years. In radio that's the golden goose and ultimate aim. It's the most prestigious slot, with the most listeners, and the one that everyone wants.

I had accidentally fallen in love with radio. I would never have imagined it would be my thing, or known how to even have started, but here I was, with Joe, desperate to learn as much about the craft as possible.

In the end, I got the breakfast gig after just three years, which is still the biggest achievement that I can name for myself. I am hugely proud of that.

Capital has always been very good to me. Richard Park has been an incredible mentor, he is a bit of an Alex Ferguson-type of character, not just because he's Scottish, but if he isn't pleased with your work you'll certainly get the famous 'hairdryer treatment' and be pulled into his office. He always speaks in football analogies too, which I obviously love and relate to. Yet he knows when to praise too, and boost someone's self-esteem. He has the ability to make me feel like Lionel Messi on the pitch, like the best player in the world.

Radio – like TV – can be hard to break into. It's a cliquey industry, and most people have gone to university and learned their craft doing loads of student radio. So I wasn't taking that regular path as I clearly hadn't done either of those things.

But I kept pushing. I wanted to do well, I was hungry and ambitious.

People ask if it's very 'back stabbing' but isn't every industry a little bit? Radio can be tough, I won't lie. I wouldn't say it was cut-throat, exactly, but you have to be pretty brutal and a bit pushy.

Every other week I was knocking on the boss's door saying, 'I'm better than that person' or, 'I can make this show better.'

You have to be honest, even if there's someone else doing the show, even if that person is your friend. If you want it, and you know you can do it, you've got to go for it.

I think some feathers were ruffled as Joe and I had become a unit, we were the cool kids at the station, proving ourselves, and I think some people were jealous. You have to be like that if you want to get on. You've got to create those opportunities yourself when it comes to your career.

####

> **'Some of Joe's ideas were genius and weird – like how quickly can Nicole Scherzinger milk a goat?! He could reel anyone in with his natural charm. 'It'll totally be fine' he'd cry'**

####

No one owes you that opportunity to have a better radio show or a better TV show. If I go to a commissioner at a TV channel, I sure as hell have to go in there with a better idea than what they've currently got. You can't sit there and go, 'Can you please give me a show?'

It doesn't work like that.

You have to prove you have a better one.

For a while we carried on just doing one show a week, that graveyard Sunday slot. But Joe and I had big ideas. We'd proved ourselves, we were pulling in the numbers and the station then gave us the Saturday show, 5pm-8pm.

That was a horrendous slot for a show, everyone knows that is dog shit territory because, on a Saturday night, people aren't listening to the radio, they're going out for early drinks and those types of things. But I didn't care. 'Give me the show!' I said. We took it, and also happily landed the Sunday 9pm-12am slot.

We pretended to ourselves that our Sunday morning show was the biggest show on the station. Because we were young, we knew all the things that were going on YouTube and Twitter and all those social media types of things. It felt like we could relate to young people, we were the same age, and we could bring fresh ideas and change the pace a bit.

We started a thing called 'Sunday selfies', which was basically getting listeners to share their lives and send in their pictures of silly things in the morning. We just tried different things.

Because it was a rubbish slot, I think the bosses were more easily persuadable into letting us try different things. We'd say, 'Look, if it works it works, if it doesn't, take it off me.'

Because I was mates with various YouTubers I thought, 'Let's get them on the show and we'll play some games, have a bit of fun with it.' It went really well, we were building our relationship with the listeners and soon Joe and I were getting the highest weekend numbers ratings Capital had ever seen. We'd go into the quarterly meetings, when you find out about audience figures, and it was such a buzz.

People seemed to be loving our vibe.

We started getting big names to come onto the show – before then there hadn't been interviews on the Sunday show.

One of my first artist interviews was with Sam Smith. It was a big deal. I was nervous, Joe used to laugh at me because I got so nervous. He said he'd be on 'neck watch' as mine would always turn bright red. I even came up in hives.

I'd known Stormzy a bit from Twitter so I asked him on the

show and he did one of his first ever radio interviews with us in 2016. That was a coup.

When Craig David announced he was making a comeback track, his first new song in years, we got him on the show. We were so excited. I remembered all the times Harley and I had listened to him as a kid. And we got Craig David rapping freestyle, which ended up going viral.

We were having a ball. We'd go to a film junket and I'd be chatting to some of the biggest stars on the planet, like Daniel Craig or Tom Cruise.

I had an absolute blast with Denzel Washington one time. He got me doing impressions of him, which he bloody loved. What a legend.

But not all the celebrities liked our style.

A certain cast member from Game of Thrones clearly hated us and I wound up stopping the interview early, it was so painful. I also once turned up to a Jennifer Lawrence junket as a superfan for a prank and revealed a tattoo of her face on my chest – it went a bit wrong as I've never seen an interview get cut off like that in my life!

Joe was always beside me at these things, getting the content in the can.

Next came the Capital Evening Show which was weeknights from 7pm-10pm.

We were a bit naughty and didn't always follow the rules.

You aren't allowed to have food or drinks in the studio, yet Joe would come in carrying two plates, knives and forks and set up a table for a three-course meal! Or we'd order a Nando's. We sometimes stuck the football on. Bit cheeky.

And once we started playing beach volleyball while live on air. We got all competitive and kept playing for 25 minutes, which meant that the emergency system which goes straight to playing songs kicked in. The bosses weren't happy about that, it was all caught on CCTV. We must have been irritating, I can see that now!

But if one of the bosses told us off or were pissed off about something, we'd just use it as material, we'd turn into something funny and talk about it on the show.

We were soon hanging out all the time, not just at work. We loved watching football together, and at weekends we'd end up in a nightclub called Tape in Bond Street, having some shots and beers.

I'm not a big fan of nightclubs myself, but Joe would say, 'We've got to go and meet the celebrities to get them on the show!'

And he was right. A lot of the artists that we'd interviewed that week would be there hanging out. So we then started making friends with them and making the next interview even better. And suddenly all these big artists were actually requesting to do our shows. The bookings team were delighted, though it caused some awkwardness at times if people were asking to come on our show instead of someone else's.

Some of Joe's ideas were genius and weird – like how quickly can Nicole Scherzinger milk a goat?! I've no idea how, but Joe managed to persuade Nicole to do it. He would be that person who could convince anyone to get behind an idea. He could reel anyone in with his natural charm.

'It'll totally be fine,' he'd cry with great confidence. And it normally was. However mad the concept, he'd somehow find a way to execute it.

We had this one idea of doing Cab Roulette. So there would be a celebrity in a car with me – someone like James Cordon –

and I'd ask them questions, and if they didn't want to answer it (I remember he wouldn't tell me who his worst guest on Carpool Karaoke had been) then we'd stop the cab and let some random stranger hop in for a ride.

This was classic Joe. Nothing was unachievable. One time I said to him, 'I want to do a show in space!'

I don't know how he did it, but sure enough he had me talking to an astronaut on the International Space Station. Sometimes it backfired, Joe was actually banned from the steel drum community once for hiring steel drum bands, promising them things and not doing it.

But we were having fun, and attracting bigger names each week.

Meghan Trainer, Ariana Grande, Selena Gomez, Dua Lipa, big American artists came on to our shows. And we were getting them to do fun stuff, it felt like we were hanging out with the artists, not just 'talk to me about the song'. We wanted to make them feel special. The nice thing now is if I watch old interviews back, I can still hear Joe in the background laughing or clapping because we were just on the same vibe.

It was a huge moment for us when we got Justin Bieber coming to Capital. Because there were two breakfast shows, Marvin Humes used to do the main interviews and then we got the scraps normally, when celebrities had got a little tired of promoting, and we'd have to wake them up.

But when Capital bosses said 'we've only got time to do one interview with Justin Bieber and we want you guys to do it', we knew it was a big, big deal for us.

And it was the weirdest scenario we'd been in so far with the Justin interview. He was actually wheeled in on a big TV screen rather than being in person.

Now of course we're all used to seeing Zoom interviews thanks to the pandemic, but at the time it felt very odd.

We were sitting in the studio and that was the first time there was a lot of press in the room as well as just our gang. People were taking pictures and the big bosses came down to watch us, it was all a bit of a kerfuffle with so many people there.

But the interview went well. I think by 2017 the station then realised we were good and deserved a better platform.

####

> **'It was Ed Sheeran who dropped me in it. He's a mate and we talk to each other loads so I'd told him in confidence I'd been given the job. But bless Ed, he's such a great one for bigging up his friends'**

####

I was dominating at the station and seemingly outperforming people I'd always looked up to. Lisa Snowdon had recently left, and Dave Berry was doing the breakfast show. Dave is a great guy and was always so nice to me. I can't speak on his behalf but I think he wanted to leave. I suspect he'd looked over his shoulder and saw me and Joe keen and eager and thought he didn't want to compete. I never had a conversation with Dave about it though. It's just the nature of the game, isn't it?

If someone says to you, 'What do you want to be?' what's the point of me saying, 'I want to be a middle-of-the-road radio presenter'? Of course I don't. I want to be the best presenter in the world. Otherwise, what's the point?

ROMAN KEMP – ARE YOU REALLY OK?

It was awkward at some of the ratings meetings where it was clear we were absolutely killing the numbers. People at the station had to stand up and give us a round of applause and stuff, and while I'm not normally someone who gets embarrassed, I was a bit embarrassed by that. I think people knew we were heading in the direction of the breakfast show. There were rumours that it was happening for a while, but I daren't believe them.

A few weeks after the Justin Bieber chat I was called into a meeting and told the breakfast show was ours. I came out feeling a bit shaky and not taking it all in. I'd wanted this badly, but I was expecting it would take much longer to reach this point. It didn't feel real.

Joe and I were overjoyed – it felt like we'd been knocking on the door for a long time. And now we were being rewarded. But we weren't allowed to tell anyone for a while, it was all top secret, they hadn't told Dave yet, and it was awkward.

It was Ed Sheeran who dropped me in it. He's a mate and we talk to each other loads so I'd told him in confidence I'd been given the job. But bless Ed, he's such a great one for bigging up his friends.

We went to interview him backstage – me and all the Capital crew – for a quick chat before he had a gig.

Just before we went on air he couldn't help but be excited as he greeted me.

'MATE!' he grinned. 'HUGE congratulations on getting the breakfast show.'

Everyone sort of looked at each other awkwardly.

'Oh,' said Ed. 'I wasn't supposed to know that, was I?'

We had to jump straight on with the show. Afterwards, I just said to the gang, 'You didn't really hear that, did you?'

THE BIG LIST OF MY LIFE

Finally, it was all officially announced in April 2017, and I started in May alongside a new presenter Vick Hope.

I really felt like I'd made it. My ambition had paid off. But with success comes pressure, and there were some rocky times ahead.

MY DARKEST HOUR

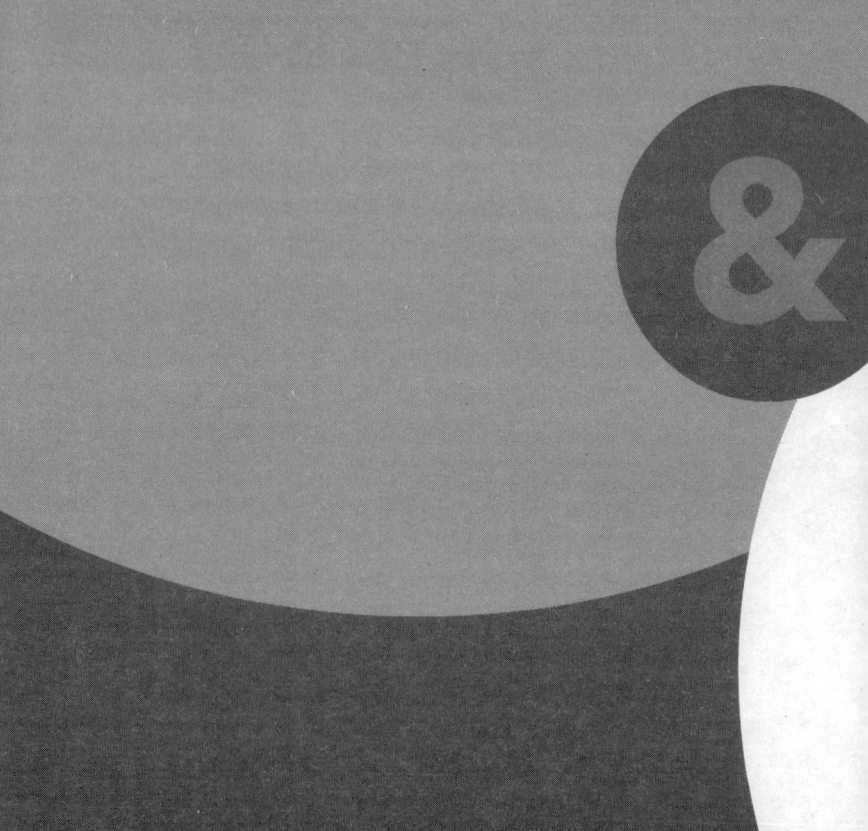

PART 3.

BRIGHTER DAYS TO COME

ROMAN KEMP – ARE YOU REALLY OK?

Until Joe's death two years ago I never imagined I'd be telling everyone about the pills I take or speaking so openly about my mental health. It's not something I thought I'd be shouting about. I was afraid of putting it out there.

Because I'm a so-called 'celebrity', with a nice flat in central London, a fun job, great mates, and come from a very loving family, I shouldn't 'have' depression, right?

That's what I told myself for years. I felt embarrassed that I should have any problems. Like I didn't have the 'right' to be feeling very low at times. Some people have genuinely hard lives. I realise that I am blessed with good fortune.

'What's HE got to moan about, eh?'

That's what I thought people would say if I dared to talk about this. And I wouldn't blame them.

But my life isn't all glossy premieres, joking on-air and hanging out with famous people. It hasn't been plain sailing, plenty of times I've found myself curled up in a ball crying with despair.

Another thing that worried me about talking about my depression was that everyone would think I was a fraud. Because every morning, by 6am, I'm sitting in my radio booth at work, playing happy pop songs, being all jokey, smiley, trying to entertain people and make them laugh. I'm the cheerful radio guy! I bring the fun and sunshine to people's mornings! That's what I'm paid to do for a living. And that's not some fake act. That's my job. I absolutely love it, grafted to get it, and don't get me wrong, I know how lucky I am to have it.

So I was concerned that speaking about my mental health struggles would harm my career, and make people think I was a fake. Lying to them on air every single day.

I was also put off about seeming 'unstable', in case bosses

didn't want to hire me in the future or saw me as being flaky, unreliable and mental. My mum Shirlie – my biggest supporter in life – was also a little hesitant about me telling the truth. 'Really, Ro?' she said, worried it would seriously affect my career. 'Are you sure this is the right thing to do?'

I wasn't sure, to tell the truth. In fact, I felt shit-scared because for many years I've kept quiet about the fact that each day I take a drug called sertraline, which is a common antidepressant and anti-anxiety pill.

I was 15 when I was first diagnosed with depression. I'm turning 30 next year, so that's half my life I've been taking little so-called happy pills.

It just helps me feel more… normal.

As I've explained, it was Mum who initially noticed something had changed in me. It wasn't because my life had changed. No bad thing or trauma had happened to alter my behaviour. But she arranged for me to speak to the doctors. They did various tests as well as speaking to me about how I was feeling. Then they confirmed my diagnosis of chemical depression.

People can have depression for many, many reasons. In my case, I wasn't releasing enough serotonin.

Serotonin, as you might already be aware, is a chemical messenger that's believed to act as a mood stabiliser. It's thought to help us sleep and boost our sense of natural wellbeing. With chemical depression, the serotonin levels aren't reaching the peaks that the average person has and some people, like me, just need a little bit of extra help to get them functioning like normal.

The first pill I was put on at 15 was 50 mg of Fluoxetine a day.

It's an SSRI antidepressant (which stands for Selective Serotonin Reuptake Inhibitors) and how these work is by blocking the reabsorption of serotonin into the nerve cell that released it. Effectively, it means that the serotonin acts for longer on your brain and body.

After seven years on that, I was told that actually, Fluoxetine can increase the incidence of suicidal thoughts, so I was taken off that. Please don't panic if you are taking this drug – I am not a doctor, I just take the advice. What wasn't right for me might work well for you because there are so many variants at play.

I was then put on one called Citalopram, as doctors believed it would suit me better. It left me feeling really spaced out so it wasn't for me, but again, it's one of the most prescribed ones so people have different reactions.

Then, when I was 24, I was put on 100 mg of sertraline a day. And that's what I still take now.

With any long-term medication though, the doctors will review it every few months to check you're receiving the right dose and to keep an eye on how it's working for you. There are new developments in drugs all the time, so it's important to keep reviewing it all with your GP, and don't forget to keep checking in with yourself, too. You know yourself better than anyone, after all.

I know from experience these pills work for me. Massively.

But with all medication, there are risks of side effects. For me personally they can make me feel a little more fatigued and I sometimes wonder if they stop me feeling some of the 'highs' in life as well as stopping the awful 'lows'.

One of the things I find is that the pills stop me from being able to cry. You might think, 'so what?'

But sometimes I feel I actually want to have a good old

cry and experience that release of emotions. I recently walked around the whole of Primrose Hill willing myself to have a cry because I was having a shit time. So there are times when I get frustrated with that.

And there have been occasions when I've stopped taking them. I can have a little bit of a self-destructive side to my character. It's like wanting to test myself, seeing how bad I feel without them. Like holding your breath under water to test yourself when you're a kid.

I worry about admitting this. But having spoken to many other guys with depression since I've been honest about it all, I've realised I am not the only guy who does this.

But I have learned that it's stupid not to take them.

The time when I reached my lowest point, and had thoughts of taking my own life (which I'm coming to), was one of those times when I'd stopped taking my pills for a week.

Seeing how that turned out made me see why it's important to keep taking them.

If for any reason I've come off my tablets – whether being self-destructive or simply forgetting to pack them if I've gone away – my whole demeanour changes. I'll trundle along fine for five days, maybe 10, but then I've gotten out of this cycle and it catches up with me.

I don't like the person I become. People close to me can often tell and will ask whether I've remembered to take them.

There's always been a lot of stigma around taking antidepressants. But why is it so much more acceptable to talk about our physical health, yet not our mental wellbeing?

If you break your leg, you go and get it fixed up by the doctors, right? There's no shame in that. And if a guy is going to the gym and thinks, 'I'm gonna get really big, I want to bulk up on protein powders,' they'll openly ask their mate for tips and discuss which protein powder they're on.

How I see it now is that taking antidepressants is just like the guy in the gym taking protein powder, but it's benefitting my brain instead of my body. I want to be at that normal level of happiness so I can live my life. I'm trying to do what I can to make sure that I can lift those weights mentally.

I also take vitamin D every day, and have the occasional shot of vitamin B12, which is supposed to help keep your body's blood and nerve cells healthy. For some reason, I always have it in my head that how I will die eventually is from a heart attack. So I try to do what I can to stay healthy.

I find that taking antidepressants helps stop me from worrying about all the things that are in my head, because some days that worry just takes over everything. It gets too much for me.

My best way of describing depression is that it's like your brain has Mike Tyson inside it, it just beats you up – left hook, jab, cross – and there's nothing you can do to defend yourself properly as you've never had a single boxing lesson in your life. You feel like you just can't do anything except take it. Punch after punch after punch as you're curled up in a corner, helpless against your angry Mike Tyson brain.

Not every day is this bad, of course, some days are better than others. Some days are trouble-free and even brilliant, but when you get in a bad place, it can be lonely and dangerous and very, very dark.

Sadly, depression is not something you can make go away altogether by just taking pills. The doctor doesn't hand them over saying, 'Here's a cure, it'll be gone forever now.'

It's something you learn to deal with. You'll learn to know

there are going to be times when it's really tough, and then there are going to be times when it's okay and you feel great.

It's just about how you educate yourself and how you deal with the tough moments.

Not everyone suffers with their mental health. And if you're one of those lucky ones, I'm glad for you. But check in on your friends.

I don't want kids to grow up feeling ashamed if they're having a bad time. They shouldn't be keeping it a secret.

Not everyone who suffers depression will feel pills are the answer. But whatever works for you – some people prefer to go in and sit with a therapist and pour their heart out, or some people prefer meditation. Some people prefer just to go to the gym, it's all about coping mechanisms.

I've tried them all, and learned that taking pills massively helps me. It's like a tool box and you need to try different things to know what works for you. What will give you those boxing gloves, power and techniques needed in the ring when your brain decides to come and pick a fight with you?

One summer's day in Brixton, 2019

In hindsight, I think one of the many reasons why I was so angry at Joe, after he'd gone, was because he never spoke to me about just how shit he was feeling. There was never any inkling this could happen.

It was such a shock. If I had lined up 20 of my mates in a row (well, if I had 20, which I don't) and had been asked to put them in order of who I believed was most likely to ever take their own life, I would honest to God have put Joe right at the back of that queue.

He had no history of poor mental health. Unlike me. And Joe knew full well that I had suffered my own thoughts about suicide only the year before his death. I had told him about this – why did he not feel he could come to me if he had been having similar thoughts?

It was the summer of 2019 when I hit my own very lowest time.

I'd been on the Capital Breakfast show for three years by now, and I'd just agreed that I'd go on the hit ITV series I'm A Celebrity… Get Me Out Of Here later that year. I've loved the show since I was a kid and I was thrilled to be asked.

It felt the right time for me. I'd carved out a career for myself on radio and wouldn't just be there as 'Martin Kemp's kid', a label that has brought me mixed feelings all my life.

But it felt a big deal, exposing myself on telly like that to all the nation. And the decision to do it was giving me a fair amount of anxiety, too.

I was working out hard at the gym in preparation. But I was going through this kind of back-and-forth over whether or not I should be doing the show. Putting myself out there. Encouraging judgement, which I've honestly feared all my life. It was making me nervous.

I was also going through new contract negotiations with Capital and I was trying to move house. I was living in Brixton at the time, I had a girlfriend and a dog, and I was having some stressful issues with a neighbour. Perhaps these issues seem silly to other people, and I'm sorry if that's the case. But these were still the problems I felt I had that were causing me real angst.

When I got back from work one day, I felt low, anyway, and then I saw I had a tax bill come through that was for more money than I thought it would be. I could still cover it, I was good for the cash, but it was a relatively new and 'adult' thing getting to grips with being freelance and dealing with tax returns. All these little normal life stresses suddenly felt overwhelming to me at that time.

On top of it all, as I say, I was going through a bit of a self-destructive period and I hadn't taken my antidepressant tablets for a week. Stupid, I know.

Basically, I had all these things on my mind.

And that particular day, it felt like anything in my head that could have been a problem, was a problem. Have you ever had that feeling when you're hungover, and the next day you have this paranoia, where stuff just makes you feel a little bit edgy?

It was like that – but a million, zillion times worse. It was like being caught out by my own brain about everything. A horrible, negative zone where my inner psyche just spiralled in a big, messy, ugly blur.

I got in the shower, came out and just had my pants on, it was a hot summer's day.

If you've seen the Jim Carrey film Me, Myself & Irene, you'll know his character Charlie has schizophrenia. And he lets people walk all over him, suppressing his anger, and then all of a sudden – BOOM! – he just snaps.

There's a scene where Jim Carrey just dives into this new personality, a second character called Hank. And I felt exactly like that at that moment. All of a sudden, it was as if a second version of Roman had dived into me. My head was going round and round with stuff that wasn't even logical.

How was I doing at work?

Am I only doing my job because of who my dad is?

Am I being a good boyfriend?

Have I paid my tax bills?

Do I look bad?

Am I ever going to achieve anything?

All these pressures came on top of me and at me from all sides. All I know is that I was in my house and I was in my pants, crying, and I couldn't stop worrying about everything.

I'd just had enough. And I just wanted to stop the stress.

I didn't really know what to do with myself. The only thing I could do was drop down to the floor on my knees, with my hands around my head, and just cry and cry.

And from about 11am in the morning until about two in the afternoon, I sat down on the floor and cried. All these things in my life felt completely overwhelming, like they were constantly punching me in the head. I simply felt like 'this ain't for me, this life'.

My mind just kept circling.

What's the point of me? Why am I carrying on?

And at that point, the only thing I could think was, 'well, I'll just take my life. I'll kill myself'. Because, honest to God, that felt like the only way to stop this hopeless feeling.

I can't do this anymore. I can't keep getting hit.

I remember searching on my phone, looking for timetables for trains.

I thought, 'it's a 10-minute walk away to the station. I'll just make sure I go to the very front or the very end so that no one can even see me do it. I'll go to the train station, I'll step onto the track. I'll just jump in front of the train.'

I felt so worthless, consumed with self-hatred and loathing. I wanted it all to go away. For life to stop and for me to slip into oblivion.

I felt a weird sense of what I can best describe as relief that I could choose to do that. Just end it. Because when the rest of your life feels out of control, taking your own life is the one thing you can still control.

For the next hour it was like I was gearing myself up to do it.

Do I talk to my parents? Do I see this though? Do I let them know?

And it was when I was staring at my phone looking at the train timetables that my mum rang.

I don't know why she rang me. It was just by chance.

But my phone was ringing and Mum's name and face was on the screen.

I stared at it for a few rings and then I picked it up.

I was sobbing non-stop. I wasn't making any sense at all. It's all very blurry what I can remember. But I could hear all these noises in the background. This is classic Mum, she's always moving around when I'm on the phone. I always think, 'Just fucking sit down, woman!'

But I could hear the dogs barking and the sound of Mum getting into the car, and then the phone got passed quickly to my sister Harley, sitting in the passenger seat. Mum had told her to keep me talking while she was driving and not let me hang up.

And they set off from the family home in Hertfordshire and drove to my house at the time in Brixton, south London. For an hour Harley just talked to me, constantly. I really couldn't tell you what she was saying, just silly stuff to distract me I think.

I didn't admit to her then what I had been really thinking about the train tracks. Or what I'd been planning to do.

Mum had seen me in bad states before. She'd seen me being low and tearful. And she sensed this time especially was not good. Her instincts told her that she needed to get to me. And she was absolutely right.

Mum and Harley arrived within the hour and came into the house with the dogs. I remember from the window seeing the car pull up outside and I was still only wearing my pants. We must have hugged, but I can't remember what we talked about. I still didn't tell them what I'd been planning. They stayed for a few hours, until I calmed right down.

It's a very strange place to be. They call it a mental breakdown for a good reason, because your whole mind breaks down and everything goes blank afterwards. But I must have got into bed that night and got up for work the next day and carried on.

Mum has always been so good with me. I've always been a sensitive kid and she's always been there for me. Supportive, nurturing, reassuring. I know I am so lucky.

It wasn't until I made Our Silent Emergency, a few months after Joe's death, that I ever admitted to Mum just how bad I had been that day in Brixton.

That was the first time I told her the truth, on a walk at Chorleywood Common. We cried and hugged and she thanked me for being honest.

My dad was equally unaware of just how bad that situation had been. As far as he knew, I was simply in a bad place and that I'd had a bit of a wobble.

When I finally opened up I felt relieved to have been totally transparent with them. Sharing the truth is not easy sometimes, but you do feel lighter. I'm so glad I had that conversation with my family.

Now, I feel embarrassed about the whole incident. I feel angry with myself that I nearly did that. That I could have upset and destroyed the happiness of everyone I love by taking my own life.

But I have to tell people and admit I was there. I was the

person in that dark place. One in five people consider taking their lives at some point, and on that day in 2019, I was one of them.

After that episode, I started seeing a brilliant therapist for a while. Everyone has to before they go on I'm A Celebrity, I suppose it's to make sure you're in the right state of mind. They need to know you're OK and want to give you the chance to talk about your problems. I was actually really lucky because it was the perfect chance to sort myself out.

Therapy is great and I've certainly used it at times in my life when I've needed to. For me it's a useful tool, and I will use that plus my tablets as part of the armour I sometimes need to protect my mental health. I see it like it's an extra bit of ammo against my brain when I need it.

If you've never tried therapy, you might be put off by the idea it's all about lying on a leather couch and telling a stranger your darkest secrets and then they tell you what to do. But it's not that at all. Or it doesn't have to be that.

I do have to admit, though, that I lied in some of those sessions to my therapist. She was so fantastic I have some guilt about that. But I felt like if I was totally honest about having those suicidal thoughts, they would say I was too vulnerable to do the show.

Understandably, they have to prioritise people's mental wellbeing and welfare, so I kept that part of my life out of the sessions. I've sometimes wanted to go back and tell her how brilliant she was for me, to let her know how much she helped me and that I'm sorry I lied but that I wanted to do the show.

Therapy for me helped me realise how much control I have. How I can change the way I feel. It made me see that my feelings are up to me, they're not up to anyone else.

It helped me with many things, like if I see trolls online or people send me tweets saying I'm shit, I don't get upset. I can't let that dictate my feelings. If what I'm doing is still making me happy, then that's all that matters.

For me, the therapist's room was a safe place to ask myself the questions I needed to.

I always see it like you have to get from A to B. You're doing the driving. All they're doing is pulling the steering wheel, but it's you who has the foot on the gas.

It's such an empowering place where you make your own decisions. And I came out of it feeling like, 'Fuck, I am in control of my life.' That's what it did for me. It made me realise how much control over things I do have.

I know this 'lack of control' feeling is a real issue for people who are considering taking their own life. When I do my talks about suicide prevention, the majority of the audience is men, and this is what I hear time and again. I constantly find myself reminding them that they do have control. But it took talking therapy to get myself to this place.

Mum's story

Because it was Mum who first noticed the signs of depression in me, and because she's been such a massive support to me in all matters mental health, I thought it would be nice to let her have some words here, starting with when she first noticed some changes in me when I was a teenager:

> 'With Roman I could see how his behaviour had changed and how moody he'd become. Because he'd so clearly gone from being one of the funniest kids, with

a fantastic sense of humour, and someone who would constantly be trying to make everyone laugh with his impressions and songs and dances… to someone very quiet and withdrawn. It was like he didn't want to give anything of himself to other people, he'd become disconnected and disassociated from the rest of the family.

For my 50th birthday we went to Dubai and Ro was very withdrawn. We kept saying, 'Come to breakfast, come and join us all,' but the mornings were the worst time for him.

It was only later, after he'd been to see the doctor, and I really asked what they had talked about, when Roman described how bad he felt.

'When I wake up in the morning,' he admitted. 'I feel like something really dreadful has happened.'

He'd never told me that before, but it broke my heart because I recognised that exact feeling myself, from when my own hormones were out of whack at times in my life. It feels like you have got physical knots inside you, like something is pushing you down, but you don't know why.

I felt so sad for Roman.

I recognised the pattern in my dad, I'd grown up with his depression and his grumpiness all my childhood. My dad would never say if he felt low, he would never say he had depression. He just got moody and grumpy and aggressive with his family.

I've always been overly empathetic, so I really quickly pick up on people's energy and I'm very sensitive to it.

What I was really concerned about is that people with depression can turn to alcohol to try and make them feel better. It was really common growing up where I lived in Bushey, where a lot of the dads would come home drunk and start attacking their wives.

So the main thing I felt when Roman was given antidepressants was relief – that it might stop him from turning to self-medication in that way down the line. I knew I didn't want my kids smoking dope or boozing heavily. I wasn't going to allow that to happen.

With Roman I think it really helped that I could explain he was feeling depressed because it was his chemical imbalance and his hormones. The more you can talk to someone and explain why they may be feeling like they do and that they don't necessarily have control over it, it can help them understand that feeling horrible isn't their fault.

Within just a week of Roman taking antidepressants, I could see the change. It wasn't that he overnight became the happiest person ever, but it was more like having my boy back again. His fun-loving personality returned, he was once again making us laugh and enjoying himself and loved time being with his family again. It made me realise just how low he must have been before.

I don't claim to be an expert on depression or dealing with loved ones suffering from it. But from my own experiences I developed tips that worked for Roman and me. Using any opportunity I could to really check in with how he was feeling. Often the car was the best place, with me driving and focused on the road he would start blurting out the things that were on his mind. This trick also worked on long dog walks – as well as getting some exercise, which is a long-proven mood-booster.

Never try to raise an important discussion over dinner. Food should be something you're enjoying and nourishing yourself with now. I had a friend when I was younger whose father we only saw at mealtimes, when he'd lecture us and ask questions. I would get so nervous of him that I didn't want to eat, then was told to eat it all up, which is the last thing you want to do when you're feeling anxious. I firmly believe food should be something to be enjoyed at leisure for your nourishment. So I've learned never to bring up heavy conversations at the dinner table with the family. That's not the right time for a heart to heart.

Try to encourage gratitude every day. It's easy to learn this one from pets. When you leave a dog and it hasn't seen you for 10 minutes, it's so excited because time is irrelevant to them and they're just happy and grateful to see you.

Instead of waking up and thinking, 'What have I got to do today?' or how you can push yourself to achieve (which I'm guilty of and I know Roman can be too), try to wake up and think about the things you really appreciate – whether it's your family, your home, friends you love or the football you've just played. Otherwise you don't appreciate things until they're gone. I learned this the hard way myself after losing people I loved. Now I try to be more aware.

Find different ways of forming intimacy. I love going over to Roman's flat and helping him tidy up or organise his wardrobe. I find that being able to do mundane chores together, like folding laundry or rearranging things, gives us an opportunity to chat about silly little things which can help me gauge how he really is doing. These small, everyday interactions can lead to some lovely moments together.

Get advice from as many different kinds of people as you can.

If your child or a loved one has any kind of mental health diagnosis, read as much as you can and speak to as many different people as you can. Really do your research – not just by asking medical people.

Everyone is different in terms of what helps them, and people don't necessarily shout about their mental health, so you need to be open about your own as well as curious about different opinions and tips. You never know, your hairdresser might have some brilliant advice.

People ask me if I am very proud of Roman, or surprised by his success.

In truth, I always had high expectations of him. He's always had a different perspective on life.'

Shirlie

Brighter days to come...

People always ask me where I want to be in five years' time. I find that hard to answer. When you're living with depression it's often better to live in the here and now.

Looking too far ahead and setting yourself targets can ramp up your anxiety.

When I think back to the last five years, I wouldn't have believed most of the things that have happened to me. So I know how impossible it is to predict much of this crazy life.

MY DARKEST HOUR & BRIGHTER DAYS TO COME

Will I still be doing my radio show in five years? Who knows? Some hot young jock will come along, and they'll want them and not me. And that's understandable, that's what this job is. It's all about being relevant. And once you lose that, it's time to move on. If you don't understand that, then you're in the wrong industry.

These days my hopes for the future aren't ever about my career really.

My hopes for the future are all about what I want to happen in my personal life. And what I really want in my personal life, what I long for, is to become a dad in the next five years. More than anything else.

I don't see myself with a gaggle of kids, three maximum would be all I could handle, and of course I'll want one of them to be the best footballer in the world – but with my genes that's a tall order!

I do worry that they might suffer from depression, like I have. But I also know I would be well placed to see the signs and I hope I would be well experienced enough to help them. Like my mum was with me.

I am very vocal about the fact we need to do more to equip our kids to talk about their feelings and understand their moods and have the confidence to admit when they're struggling. I've learned so much in the past couple of years about why it's important to address mental health early on. I will certainly be going into my kids' schools one day to ask about what tools they are equipping youngsters with to deal with their emotions.

Like my parents did with me, I'll be supporting them with whatever they want to do in life, whether that's the entertainment industry or not. Most importantly, I'll just want them to be themselves.

My whole life has never been about chasing fame, or chasing money. It's about chasing happiness.

First of all, though, I have to meet someone! Please wish me luck. I'm on dating apps, like everyone is nowadays. But I also love meeting new people organically. I don't mind how I meet someone, and I don't care what they do. The only thing that matters is the connection I have with someone. I am ready for the next person I meet to be the person I want to spend the rest of my life with.

And in 10, 15 or 20 years down the line I dream about being settled down and living out of the limelight. Perhaps I'll be abroad, learning about new cultures and places, and being taught new things.

I know now that my depression won't miraculously go away. And I won't stop taking my pills. Even if they turned out to be a total placebo, I know that they work for me. But I think I am now in better control of my depression, because I am accepting of it. I am accepting that there are days where I won't feel good. I will have calm periods of two or three months, then I might go into a little mental low, or black spot.

It's a little bit of a cycle with me. And I don't know whether it's something that triggers it, but it seems to happen once every two or three months. I'll just have a day when I'll be in that zone. The more I'm accepting of that, aware of it and curious about it, I can say to myself, 'This is normal, and it's absolutely fine to feel this way sometimes.'

I've learned rather than fight it, it can be better to almost indulge myself in those feelings… and know that they will pass. Give myself permission to experience the lows, and show myself kindness.

Guys can be terrible for doing that, but it does help.

MY DARKEST HOUR & BRIGHTER DAYS TO COME

If I feel a mood descending, it can help to recognise and label the emotions. To make a plan to see a friend or be with someone I love. To go back and walk the dogs at my mum's house and have long chats with her. Or to watch a film or just relax and to try and find some time for me.

I step away from social media, I switch off my phone and I try to remember all the things I am grateful for. I try to write gratitude lists as it can help seeing it on paper. My mum is very big on the importance of gratitude, and the older I get the more I understand why this is right. Now she's been baptised, and is more interested in Christianity, she talks more about the role of forgiveness too. We've had some really deep and meaningful chats about this.

As the second anniversary of Joe's death loomed in August I became fearful something bad would happen again.

In my head I was dreading it. Almost like having a PTSD-like anxiety. I found myself having flashbacks.

Mum encouraged me to talk about the nerves I was feeling, and then to hand them over to something bigger than me. Whether that is God or the universe, it helped to have faith in something bigger.

So on the second anniversary of Joe's death, I wrote to him, and told him how I felt.

This is what I wrote...

Dear Joe,

How have I not heard your voice for two years? How have we not caused havoc in the studio or in some dingy Soho bar? How have I not been able to call you to tell you I love you?

> *All I want is for you to feel happy. Forever I will say that through gritted teeth, I can literally see you stood in front of me holding your hands up and saying "sorry buddy, I fucked up".*
>
> *I wish I could tell you Tottenham still haven't won anything. Tell you how incredible and strong your family have been in changing the lives of people because of something so devastating.*
>
> *You'd be so proud.*
>
> *I miss you every time I walk into the studio and don't have you by my side, every time I need someone just to tell me how I'm in the right even if I'm not.*
>
> *Every time I think about my life moving forward I fantasise about telling my kids about you, about how my best friend Joe was the type of human I want them to be.*
>
> *It hurts so much. I just want you back mate... back to how it was. Xx*

Afterwards, I had a cry. I messaged his family, and I went to bed until the day had passed.

When someone you love takes their own life, there is a lot of anger. As much as I try to be forgiving, I have not reached a point of forgiving Joe. I don't think I ever will, in all honesty. But I will always try to gain more understanding and work towards forgiveness.

When I am by myself I talk to Joe a lot, or if I have a memory of him I will tell him about it and I will tell him that I love him.

Looking back to the time when I wanted it all to end, I just feel so grateful that I was lucky enough to have loved ones around me. I am so grateful I didn't become a statistic.

MY DARKEST HOUR & BRIGHTER DAYS TO COME

As I approach turning 30, I realise how very lucky I have been to have been on this wonderful journey called life.

Through the highs and lows, I wish you love and happiness too. Stay safe and please look out for each other.

THE END OF THE BOOK

Stuff that's good to know

I wanted to put the serious facts at the back of the book so they're easy to access. Here, I'll mention a couple of books I've found really useful, explain some mental health strategies and give you a list of contact info for a few organisations.

Some of the most important lessons during my research for the BBC 'Silent Emergency' documentary were learned from meeting Professor Rory O'Connor, who leads the Suicidal Behaviour Research Lab at the University of Glasgow.

- This is one of the leading research labs in the world for understanding and preventing suicide.
- Rory is also the President of the International Association for Suicide Prevention, which is the leading suicide prevention organisation globally.
- He has been working in suicide research for more than 25 years and he told me about his own experiences of suicide bereavement when we met. He talked movingly about losing his first mentor to suicide in 2011 and also the devastation when he lost one of his best friends to suicide in 2008. He spoke about the guilt and regret that he still feels about their deaths and how he wishes he had done more to reach out to them in their hour of need.
- He said that it is this sense of failure that continues to drive him, when he gets up every morning, to do more to understand and prevent suicide.

It was fascinating seeing up-close what Rory and his team do. They work closely with people who have been suicidal, to try to make sense of the wide range of factors that lead to suicide.

One of the things he showed me in Glasgow was how his team is trying to understand emotion regulation by looking at changes in electrical activity in sweat. Although this sounds a bit surprising and you may be wondering how is this associated with suicide (I did too!), Rory explained how changes in sweat can help researchers understand changes in emotion regulation.

Emotion regulation is another term for how we feel and process emotions – and in people who are suicidal their emotion regulation doesn't seem to be working as well as it should be. He thinks that his research will lead to better markers of who may be especially vulnerable to suicide. Fascinating, right?

He also talked a lot about the complexity of the factors that can lead to suicide and about the many different psychological and social factors that increase suicide risk. He highlighted that there is no single factor that leads to suicide and that we need to look beyond mental illness explanations and to remember the social context is really important as well.

Here's what he said: 'Although depression is a risk factor for suicide, the challenge is that most people who are depressed never become suicidal. So our research is trying to work out which person with depression is most likely to become suicidal and potentially take their own life. We are trying to disentangle the combination of biological, psychological and social factors that are most risky.'

Rory's work helps us to make sense of why around 6,000 people in the UK and more than 703,000 people die by suicide each year. His team has also done a lot of work on childhood trauma, which is another factor that is important in understanding suicide risk. In some of their studies, they have found that four out of five people who attempt suicide have experienced trauma as children, and this has had a longer-term impact on their mental health and wellbeing. That reminds us of how important it is to support young people, especially now as we recover from the pandemic, when we know that so many young people's mental health was affected.

To help people understand suicide, Rory has also written an excellent and award-winning book called When It Is Darkest: Why People Die By Suicide and What We Can Do To Prevent It.

I was so impressed by the book and the work that Rory does when I met him. If you want to really understand why people end their lives, please read this book. If you want to support a friend or someone in your family who is suicidal or who has lost a loved one to suicide, this is full of helpful tips and brilliant advice. This book comes from the heart.

In it, Rory takes us on a journey of some of the people he has met who have been suicidal or who have been bereaved by suicide. He also talks about his own experience of losing loved ones to suicide, his own mental health, what the research tells us about why people die by suicide and what we all can do to reach out and support others. When I asked Professor O'Connor why people kill themselves, he said: 'Most people who die by suicide feel trapped or defeated. These feelings may also have been triggered by loss, rejection and shame. In a nutshell, those who are suicidal feel trapped by unbearable mental pain.

'It isn't that they want to die, it is that they want the pain to end. They may feel alone, depressed, have experienced trauma or have been bullied. They often feel like they're a burden on loved ones, and that others would be better off if they were dead. Sadly, they see suicide as the only option for them. It is like a perfect storm of factors coming together, when they cannot see an alternative but to kill themselves, as the ultimate way of ending their pain.'

He also talked about the importance of looking out for each other: 'Anyone can become suicidal if this perfect storm of factors comes together. That is why it is so important to check-in with your friends or family members if you are concerned about them. Always ask twice, to check that they're doing okay.'

The big S-question

'My advice is to ask someone directly if they are feeling suicidal or are thinking about ending their life. Genuinely, asking this question could be the start of a life-saving conversation,' says Professor O'Connor. 'Some people are frightened to ask the question as they fear it might plant the idea in someone's head. By way of reassurance, it WON'T and it DOESN'T. By asking the question, a friend or family member could get the help that they may so urgently need. So, please, always ask what I call the big S-question. Also, it is worth remembering that a smile, a gesture, a message, a call, just showing someone that they matter, could save a life.'

Professor O'Connor also showed me a safety plan, which is used to keep people who may be experiencing suicidal thoughts safe. He told me: 'A safety plan is a crisis plan which helps people to identify warning signs and ways to keep themselves safe. Usually, it is co-created by a mental health professional together with someone who is suicidal or in crisis; but I'd encourage everyone to make a safety plan. It is a way of planning what we might do if the going gets tough and we start to feel overwhelmed.

'A safety plan can be so important because it could stop someone acting on their thoughts of suicide. It is a way of interrupting suicidal thoughts – so that someone doesn't act on their thoughts. This is vital as we know that the things that lead someone to becoming suicidal (e.g., being trapped by mental pain) are different from those that make it more likely that they'll act on their thoughts (e.g., being impulsive or planning a suicide attempt). That is why a safety plan is so important, as it could stop someone acting on their thoughts of suicide."

Professor O'Connor also described what the safety plan involves. He started by telling me that it has six steps as he describes each of these steps in a little detail below:

The six steps of The Safety Plan

> **Step 1.** It begins with us trying to recognise the warning signs that a crisis may be developing. These could be thoughts, feelings or behaviours that seem to come before a suicidal crisis. Some people become really agitated, others cannot sleep or feel rejected. It is really useful to try to think what these warning signs might be for all of us.

> **Step 2.** In this step, it is useful to think about coping strategies. Are there things we can do to distract ourselves, or to take our mind off whatever it is that is causing our distress without contacting someone else?

> **Step 3.** If Step 2 doesn't work, are there people or places that we can call on or go to, to help distract us? These are different for everyone, but they could include a friend or a family member or going to a coffee shop or a gym. It makes sense to try to avoid places like bars and nightclubs, where alcohol or drugs might be available.

STUFF THAT'S GOOD TO KNOW

> **Step 4.** If Steps 1 to 3 are not helping, then think about people who we can ask for help. Is there someone we can call upon in a crisis? This could be a close friend or a family member, someone we feel comfortable talking to about how we are feeling or about any difficulties we're experiencing.

> **Step 5.** It is also useful to consider which professionals or organisations we could contact during a crisis. So, in Step 5, many people think of their GP, the Samaritans or another mental health professional who we can contact if we are concerned that we cannot keep ourselves safe. For this step, it is good to write down the telephone number of these professionals or organisations, so we have it to hand in a crisis. Some people either put this number into their phone or take a photo of their safety plan so that we have it to hand when we need it.

> **Step 6.** The final step of the safety plan is focused on making the environment safe. In essence, this involves removing or restricting access to the means of suicide. If we have thought about how we might end our life, it is so important to think about how we can keep the environment safe, so that if a suicidal crisis arises, we don't have ready access to the means of harming ourselves. Arguably, this is a tricky step but it could be the most important as it may prevent us – or a loved one – from acting on our thoughts of suicide.

In his book, Professor O'Connor also talked about warning signs for when someone might be suicidal, here are the things he said to look out for:

Warning signs that someone might be suicidal

Someone may be thinking of suicide if:

- They are talking about being trapped, a burden on others and feeling hopeless about the future.
- They have experienced loss, rejection or other stressful life events and are struggling to cope.
- They are sorting out their life affairs, such as giving away prized possessions or getting their will in order.
- There is an unexplained improvement in mood. This may be because they have decided that suicide is the solution to their problems.
- There are marked changes in behaviours such as sleeping, eating, drinking, drug-taking or other risk-taking behaviours.
- They have a history of self-harm or have made a previous suicide attempt.
- They are acting or behaving unpredictably or out of character.

From Rory O'Connor (2021). When It Is Darkest. Vermilion.

If you want to learn more about Professor O'Connor's work, check out his website which has lots of useful resources:

www.suicideresearch.info

STUFF THAT'S GOOD TO KNOW

The Wellness Menu – lists of 5

I already mentioned Richie Perera – the founder of Mental Health and Life – in the Drink and Drugs chapter, but he has some really helpful ways of talking about mental health, and how to understand your own more clearly.

He encourages us to each create a 'wellbeing menu', which is a collection of activities a person enjoys doing and can choose from day in, day out. You can choose from the fun, energetic or relaxing activities several times a day.

The idea behind it is to help keep your mind and body healthy and well balanced.

> *List 5 activities you are currently doing or can easily do for your wellbeing – like going for a walk, reading a book or gardening.*

> *List 5 activities you can do with a slight lifestyle change – like yoga, meditation, breath, work or cardio exercise.*

> *Your wish list. List 5 things you may have always dreamed of doing – like flying lessons or running a marathon. Maybe it can include things you wanted to do as a child, but never got around to as an adult.*

You need to aim for at least one activity from your wellbeing menu, from intensive workouts to eight solid hours of sleep and everything in between.

Avoid activities that are consumable like drinking or that require the use of the screen. You get a bonus benefit if any of the activities are connected to nature. You then place your wellbeing menu on a wall in a prominent place.

Take an hour out to do activities from your wellness menu.

Richie reminds us that our mental health needs watering everyday and that we are the CEO of our own lives – and we each deserve to live happily and healthily.

Richie Perera: Managing People In The New Normal, published by Balboa Press, due Autumn 2022.

Help! I need somebody

There are many excellent resources available if you need support. This isn't an exhaustive list and there will be other support services too, but I hope it helps. Don't hesitate to get in touch, even if you're in doubt. Nothing lost.

Samaritans

The one mental health charity everyone has heard of, and for good reason. Every ten seconds, Samaritans respond to a call for help.

You can call them 24/7 on 116 123.

You can also write to them if you prefer to have your thoughts and feeling on paper, and they will aim to respond within seven days.

Send letters to Freepost SAMARITANS LETTERS.

You can email them too, and they will reply within 24 hours jo@samaritans.org

They also have a self-help app you can download so you can record how you're feeling, understand changing patterns in your mood and get suggestions for things that could help you stay safe in a crisis.

STUFF THAT'S GOOD TO KNOW

CALM

The charity CALM Stands for Campaign Against Living Miserably, and it runs a free, confidential and anonymous helpline as well as a webchat service, offering help, advice and information to anyone who is struggling or in crisis.

The free helpline is available every day from 5pm-midnight, on 0800 58 58 58.

They also have really useful guides on their website on all sorts of topics from exam stress (we've all had that at one time or another!), relationship break-ups and erectile dysfunction – to helping loved ones struggling with their mental health and support after suicide.

www.thecalmzone.net

Heads Together

Heads Together is a mental health initiative spearheaded by The Royal Foundation of The Prince and Princess of Wales, which combines a campaign to tackle stigma and change the conversation on mental health with fundraising for a series of innovative new mental health services.

They offer resources and advice for people working with children and young people.

https://mentallyhealthyschools.org.uk

While the Mental Health At Work programme is help everyone in the workplace prioritise mental wellbeing.

www.mentalhealthatwork.org.uk

ROMAN KEMP – ARE YOU REALLY OK?

Shout

Shout is a free text messaging service which provides 24/7 support for anyone experiencing a mental health crisis.

By texting the word 'SHOUT' to 85258 you will start a conversation with a trained Shout Volunteer, who will text you back and forth, sharing only what you feel comfortable with. The aim is to help texters move from a moment of crisis to a calm state and form a plan for next steps to find longer term support.

www.giveusashout.org/get-help

Mind

Mind is a mental health charity in England and Wales offering information and advice to people with mental health problems. It also lobbies government and local authorities on their behalf. They can help with questions about mental health problems including where to get help near you, treatment options and the advocacy services available.

You can call Infoline on 0300 123 3393 (9am to 6pm, Monday to Friday, except for bank holidays).

You can email: info@mind.org.uk

Or you can write to them at: Mind Infoline, PO Box 75225, London, E15 9FS

Meanwhile their Legal line provides legal information and general advice on mental health-related law – being detained under the Mental Health Act (sectioning), mental capacity, community care and discrimination and equality.

You can call the Legal line on 0300 466 6463 (9am-6pm,

STUFF THAT'S GOOD TO KNOW

Monday to Friday, except for bank holidays). Or you can write to: Mind Legal line, PO Box 75225, London, E15 9FS

www.mind.org.uk

NHS

On NHS inform (which is a Scottish initiative) there is a useful online guide – which aims to help you find out if you could have symptoms of depression, understand more about depression and find ways to manage or overcome depression.

This guide is based on Cognitive Behavioural Therapy (CBT). CBT helps you to examine how you think about your life, and challenge negative automatic thoughts to free yourself from unhelpful thought and behaviour patterns.

www.nhsinform.scot/illnesses-and-conditions/mental-health/mental-health-self-help-guides/depression-self-help-guide

YoungMinds

YoungMinds is a mental health charity for children, young people and their parents. Their website is full of advice and information on what to do if you're struggling with how you feel.

They also have a Parents Helpline.

You can call them for free on 0808 802 5544 from 9.30am-4pm, Monday-Friday.

There is also a webchatting service if you find that easier to access.

www.youngminds.org.uk

Clic

Sharing your experiences may help to support other people too. Clic is a free UK-wide online community supporting adults with their mental health. It offers a platform to speak safely and openly about how you're feeling. There's a chance to swap tips and advice, chat about your day, or join in on a discussion forum.

Clic also has lots of mental health resources, advice and information for you to use and share and videos to learn from.

You can sign up and see the house rules on the website.

www.clic-uk.org

Alcoholics and Narcotics Anonymous

If you think you need to talk to someone about how much alcohol you're drinking, help is available – make an appointment to see your GP for advice and support.

Alcoholics Anonymous has a free helpline – 0800 9177650 – and can help you find support groups and meetings near to where you live.

Narcotics Anonymous has a free helpline on 0300 999 1212, it's open 10am to midnight daily and will be answered by a NA member.

www.aa.org
www.na.org

STUFF THAT'S GOOD TO KNOW

And last, but certainly not least, always remember how important it is to speak to the people around you...

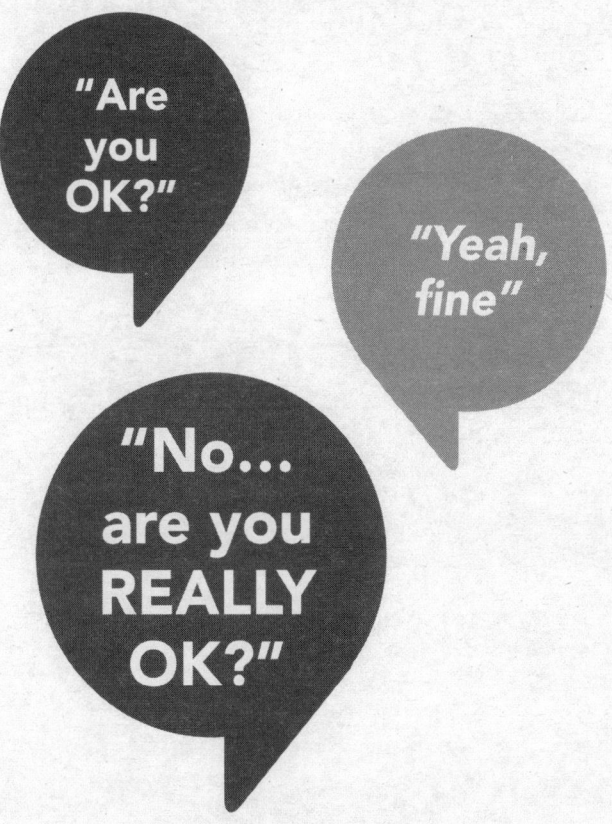

*Talk to people and get them to talk to you.
It can save lives.*